Dr. Peter Dorsen was educated at Dartmouth College, Cum Laude in classics, and the Rutgers New Jersey University School of Medicine (Newark). He has practiced general internal and sports medicine for over three decades. As a Fellow in the American College of Sports Medicine, he has served at the United States Olympic Training Center in Colorado Springs and worked as a physician with the U.S. Cross Country Ski Team. He has written over 200 human interest juried and human interest articles, and contributed to several books relating to men's issues. He is the author of the *Vikings Change the Play Against Alcohol and Other Dangerous Drugs*, *Dr. D's Handbook for Men Over 40: A Guide to Health, Fitness, Living and Loving in the Prime of Life*, *Crazy Doctor: Mixing Drugs and Mental Illness*, and *Up from the Ashes: One Doc's Struggle with Drugs and Mental Illness*. More recently, Dr. Dorsen has been a licensed alcohol and drug counsellor. He has spoken on many sports medicine and alcohol and mental health topics at US and world cross country and chemical health forums. He currently cross-country ski races at national and international master's cross country skiing races and currently takes the podium for age related win. He prides himself on his vegetarian cooking, carpentry, and gardening. He lives in Eagan, Minnesota with his partner, Nada, and their standard poodle, Saidie.

For Kata, Gabi, Bria, Nada, and my beloved parents and grandparents.

PETER J. DORSEN, M.D.

MEN OVER 60: DON'T QUIT NOW!

3·15·2023

For Jim Lafferty + family.

we're all in it together.

Peter

AUSTIN MACAULEY PUBLISHERS™

LONDON · CAMBRIDGE · NEW YORK · SHARJAH

A CIP catalogue record for this title is available from the British Library.
Copyright 2022

Cover illustration, "Resolve," by Brant Kingman and Photography by Odd Osland on the cover.

ISBN 9781398464667 (Paperback)
ISBN 9781398464674 (ePub e-book)

www.austinmacauley.com

First Published 2022
Austin Macauley Publishers Ltd®
1 Canada Square
Canary Wharf
London
E14 5AA

Those who helped me continue as a writer include my brilliant academic and eclectic cousins David Dorsen and half-a-century mentor, Professor and civil libertarian, Norman Dorsen, who, despite his incomparable erudition, accepted my New Journalism style. Jody Nolen, bless her self-destructive soul, the brilliant daughter of Dr. Bill Nolen (*The Making of a Surgeon*) was my first writing teacher who pushed me over the edge. Minneapolis Star Tribune feature writer, Ralph Thornton, who covered such minority sports as cross-country skiing and horse racing at Canterbury Downs, Minnesota, who took me under his wing but, sadly, went down in a split second with cancer. Retired University of Minnesota journalism professor, Herman Sittard, was my second writing mentor, who wisely told me, "I'd flunk anyone with a grammar or spelling error." I wish I'd listened. Dave Paulsen was there to welcome me back to cross country ski racing when I needed it most. John Kelso, Larry Geiger, Johnny Morton, and Patch Adams stood tall and supported our mutual adventure of aging.

I learned how to spell complementary medicine from the wonderfully accepting holistic medicine guru, Dr Bill Manahan, who always provided honest and supportive analyses that would serve to validate this book.

There were those who read and gave solid endorsements for my exploration of fellow men over 60. They include Peter Cleeves, Johnny Morton, Johnny, Caldwell, Ophthalmologist, Professor Dr. Edward Feinberg, Olympic physician and internist, Dr, Barry Mink, Cornell drama professor and ER MD, Dr. David Feldshuh, who wrote *Miss Evers' Boys*; Dr. Patch Adams; fellow medical School co-conspirator, Dr. Daniel Tartaglia, who, with Dr. Karen O'Neill, my New Jersey and Baltimore City Hospital comrades, were joyous participants in the social revolution of American medicine in the early seventies.

I am indebted to those who generously supported my book: minyan mate, Ron Metz; Bend Oregon fellow ski racer, Len Sher; Norwegian ski ace, Arvid Krogsveen; massage therapist to Olympians, Steve Carmazon; my MG Midget go-to guy and friend, Brad Larson; Karen Hoffrogge; and Dr. Steve Zukerman, the Roger Dangerfield of internists.

My dearest ski compadre Odd Osland systematically and unselfishly took masterly pictures for the stretching and strength chapters that are enhanced by one-time body builder, power lifter, and Colorado champion downhill skier, Doug Hagerty. My dear new son-in-law, cinematographer, Scott Kassenoff, magically created my photo for the book. He brought me Koa Blu Kassenoff, my adorable new grandson. The amazing sculptor and visual artist Brant Kingman, has again provided, "Resolve," the book cover image.

Dan Emerson, my long time editor from early writing days for *Minnesota Physician*, unselfishly read and reread versions of this book. The late Dr. Art

Leon took me under his wing for a mid-career sports medicine fellowship and an opportunity to participate in unique research. I am indebted for his foreword and continual support as the book progressed. It was my honor also to have support in many ways from the eclectic Dr. Henry Blackburn, both New Orleans jazz aficionado, and world-renowned epidemiologist.

My thoughts are always for my artistic three daughters, Bria Danielle Dorsen, Gabriella Nicole Kassenoff, and Katarina Marica Dorsen, and blessed with grandsons, Indio from "Kata" and Joey Medina, Koa Blu Kassenoff from "Gabi" and my beloved new son-in-law, Scott.

Faruk Abuzzahab, M.D., PhD, world-renowned psychopharmacologist has been my guide as well as introducing me to his lovely daughter, Nada Josephine Abuzzahab, the love of my life. My big thanks to dear friend, Louis Maravelas of "Make America Greek again" fame and his bookish love, Mary Jo Pauly. He reluctantly sold me my greatest (other) passion, a '79 MG Midget that has helped me escape the pressures from writing *Men Over 60.*

I can't forget to thank Dr. Kip Minaert, my Dartmouth soul brother, with whom I underwent dangerous but memorable ill-advised thrills and chills. I have had joy with my Duluth family, Mike Mancini and Amanda, and the now deceased Paul Maire.

Additional family members have always been in the wings: Annie Anny and their daughter, Judy Nye; "Ancha Ancha," Sanyi and Susy Gross who always provided love and understanding. I salute Dr. Seymour Lifshutz—the best internist I have ever known-and his artist wife, Phylis, who supported my writing over the years. Uncles and Aunts, Rhoda and Allan Labowitz, Uncle Bob, Aunt Rita Dorsen, and their daughter, Nan; and, especially, my beloved, Dr. Howard ("Happy") and Verna Adler, and generous with their love, Uncle and aunt, Rhoda and Allen.

But how could I ever forget my dear parents, Dr. Lydia and "Buddy" as well as incomparable grandparents, Anuka and Popuka Adler.

I have the greatest debt of gratitude to Jasmine Smith, who patiently guided me through the throes of publishing this book.

Thank you to Ethan Scurrah, for your superb rendering of the cover for *Men Over 60: Don't Quit Now!*

"Dr. Dorsen offers an antidote to time and a commitment to daily respect for your body and mind. With insight and clarity, he encourages us to make health a daily habit."

Dr. David Feldshuh, playwright, emergency physician, and Pulitzer nominee for Miss Ever's Boys based on the devious Tuskegee syphilis study. He is the retired director of Cornell Theatre.

"*Men Over 60: Don't Quit Now!* merges practical advice, inspiration, and humor in a lively read. Dr. Dorsen's medical knowledge and willingness to report on the ups and downs of his own over-60 body are unique. The book bolsters confidence, shows paths to a fulfilling later life, and provides guidance for sexual resurgence."

Peter Cleaves, Director of the Academic Center, University of Texas, and author of several books including *A Mexico Escape 1936 – Biking the Pan American Highway* (Amazon: Monee, Illinois, 2020) by Richard D. Cleaves, co-edited with Richard and Peter Cleaves.

"The ever-inquisitive Dorsen is the optimal age to write this book based on the program for success in his xc skiing. He's old enough to have experienced the slow development of xc in the US during the '50's, '60's and 70's and old enough to witness all the advancements in the available information for maintaining what I call a good lifestyle. Plenty of good tips here."

"Johnny" Caldwell, a member of the 1952 U.S. Olympic Nordic team in Oslo, is the author of five books that have popularized the sport of cross-country skiing as the as the "father" and guru of the sport. He coached five teams for the US at the 1966-72 and 1984 Olympic Games.
"*Men Over 60: Don't Quit Now!* supplies helpful information for men in their senior years who want to stay active and healthy. To share this type of information with senior men is an similar goal of Dr. Dorsen and myself. I recommend Dr. Dorsen's sequel to *Dr. D's Handbook* as a helpful guide to anyone interested in this age group."

Dr. Barry Mink, Internist and sports medicine doctor at the Aspen, Colorado Clinic, and Nordic Team physician at both the 1980 and 1994 Winter Olympics at Lake Placid and Lillehammer.

This is the best book I have read on how men can stay healthy and happy well into their 60's, 70's, and 80's. It is healthy, holy, all root words of holistic. *Men*

Over 60: Don't Quit Now! advises how to stay healthy and happy in each of these domains and THRIVE in our later years of life.

Dr. Bill Manahan, a retired family physician in his 80's, is author of *Fast and Simple ways of Eliminating Disease Without Medical Assistance* and Past-President of the American Holistic Medical Association.

Members of the USA cross-country master's association American XC Skiers enjoy the combination of witty prose and interesting science provided by *Men Over 60: Don't Quit Now!* Dr. Dorsen offers the right blend of facts and fun, plus a sprinkling of motivation to keep both athletes and non-athletes in the "best third of life." Most important of all -- not quitting!

John "JD" Downing
"JD," Editor of XC World Digest and National Director and President, World Masters XC Ski Association, and editor of XC World Digest

"In his comprehensive new book, "Men over 60, Don't Quit Now," Dr. Peter Dorsen addresses the challenges of aging from two, interconnected perspectives, that of a medical doctor and, that of a life-long competitive athlete.
As a physician, Dr. Dorsen has seen in many of his patients the negative impacts of coronary heart disease, smoking, lack of exercise, poor nutrition and even a lack of self-worth, the latter brought on by retirement. At the same time, Dr. Dorsen has been able to confront and delay these age-related challenges in his own life through his enthusiastic participation in strenuous, outdoor exercise (cross-country skiing, cycling, distance hiking), a nutritious diet, and the cultivation of a positive mental outlook."

John "Morty" Morton, two-time Olympic biathlon competitor, and three-time Olympic biathlon team leader, 20-year Dartmouth Nordic ski coach, founder of Morton Trails, and author of *Don't Look Back:, Medal of Honor: Unveiling the Agony and Ecstasy Surrounding the Olympic Dream* (1998), and *Celebrate Winter: An Olympian's Stories of a Life in Nordic Skiing (*2021)
-Thank you, Peter, for showing the possibility for a healthier world, making healthier men."

In "Men Over 60, Don't Quit Now," Dr. Dorsen provides the keys for all of us older Americans to improve the quality of whatever time we have remaining by enjoying physically active, productive, and fulfilling lives.

Dr. Patch Adams, physician, comedian, social activist, clown, founder of the Gesundheit! Institute, a Training Center and Clinic in West Virginia; and author of the book, *Patch Adams Bringing Good Health to You*, and film, *Patch*(1998), and *House Calls* (1998).

"I came to this book for the information, but I stayed for the inspiration. *Men Over 60:Don't Quit Now!* offers the inspiration to implement a healthy lifestyle as we pass into our 70s and 80s."

Dr. Edward Feinberg, Professor, and chair of vitreoretinal surgery (Emeritus), Boston University, and noted poodle skijorer.

Table of Contents

"We don't stop playing because we grow old.
We grow old because we stop playing."
–   George Bernard Shaw

Foreword

Arthur Leon, M.D., M.S.
Henry L. Taylor Professor in Exercise Science and Health Enhancement
School of Kinesiology, the University of Minnesota

And ought to know that from nothing else but thence came joys, delights, laughter, sports, sorrows, griefs, despondency, and lamentations. And by this, in an especial manner, we acquire wisdom and knowledge, and see and hear, and know what are foul and what are fair, what are bad, and what are good, what are sweet, and what unsavoury... and by the same organ we become mad and delirious, and fears and terrors assail us.

Hippocrates (460–370 BC)

Doctor Dorsen's *Men Over 60: Don't Quit Now!* is an apt sequel to *Dr D's Handbook for Men Over 40: A Guide to Health, Fitness, Living, and Loving in the Prime of Life.*

I recommend this well-written book to help middle-aged and older men (and women too!) maintain or, better yet, improve their health, physical fitness, and, hence, quality of life during the ageing process.

The author, Dr Peter Dorsen, a clinical practitioner as well as alcohol and drug counsellor, and a well-published medical writer, applies his skills to crafting *Men Over 60: Don't Quit Now!* as a follow-up to his earlier work, *Dr D's Handbook for Men Over 40: A Guide to Health, Fitness, Living, and Loving in the Prime of Life*, that targeted men over age forty. Reinforcing the relevance of this book is of the direction in which our society is maturing. The number of persons older than 60 is expected to double from 2010 to 2050, increasing from 40.2 million to an estimated 88.5 million. One wonders how this senior age explosion will affect the work force, the economy, and the health care system.

This book provides American Heart Association's Guidelines for a heart-healthy eating pattern to the featured chapter, "Nutrition: you are what you eat." He advises "let's get going and provides vital suggestions for staying in shape".

This book provides an extensive description of stretching exercises for maintaining or improving whole-body muscular flexibility. Detailed guidelines are also provided of exercises for promotion of muscular strength and cardiorespiratory fitness (CRF).

For the most efficient methods for both CRF and strength training, the author, himself a competitive athlete, recommends a circuit training program in the gym consisting of rotating between 6 to 10 machine stations for 40 to 60 minutes 3 to

5 times per week at an exercise intensity of 65% to 75% of a person's maximal heart rate which may be approximated by 220-age.

Physical activity and especially aerobic exercise of sufficient intensity and volume to increase aerobic fitness as assessed by peak V02 uptake assessed by exercise testing, has been referred to by Fiiuzza et al, as the real "Polypill".

This is based on the documented benefits of 150–180 minutes per week of even moderate-intensity aerobic activity in reducing risk of multiple major problems associated with ageing, including cardiovascular disease (CVD), type 2 diabetes, colon and breast cancer, as well as all-cause mortality.

Aerobic exercise, as he describes, has well-documented beneficial cardiovascular effect which can improve cerebral blood flow. This includes reduction of major risk factors for atherosclerosis, obesity, dyslipidaemia, hypertension, insulin resistance, metabolic syndrome, and type 2 diabetes. It also has direct anti-atherosclerotic effects, including improving vascular endothelial function. Regular exercise can also preserve and restore the elasticity of major conduit arteries during ageing.

Research, mainly observational, has identified modifiable medical conditions and lifestyle factors that can enhance and maintain cognitive capacity and reserve by lifelong learning and intellectual activities. Healthy dietary practices combined with regular physical activity can reduce the risk of CVD and for their positive effect on brain function and its blood supply.

Awareness and management of psychosocial problems as identified by the author in his chapters about retirement, spirituality, lack of identity, modifiable stressors, and personal losses implicit with ageing, are relevant for adaptation to the inevitable process of ageing. Muscle strengthening maintaining flexibility and posture-promoting exercise, as covered in several chapters in *Men Over 60*, may stabilise deleterious effects on the ageing process and improve awareness and avoidance of balance, gait, muscle spontaneity and speed but, of tantamount importance, reduce the risk and consequences of cognitively avoidable falls and traumatic brain injury (TBI).

Doctor Dorsen, from his medical perspective, outlines how important CVD risk factor such as lipid problems, hypertension, diabetes, obesity, or smoking not controlled by diet, and regular physical activity can be successfully managed with pharmacologic interventions.

In summary, this easy-to-read, meaty book provides concise healthy guidelines for helping attenuate the detrimental effects of ageing on physical fitness and for the prevention of common chronic diseases associated with ageing.

Prologue

"The secret of health for both mind and body is not to mourn the past, worry about the future, or anticipate trouble, but to live in the present moment wisely and earnestly."

Buddha

I am writing a handbook for men who are of retirement age. Why does society expect us to dry up and blow away? Like me, some of my friends go kicking and struggling accepting the inevitable milestone of 60. It is like it snuck up on us. The years from our forties raced by. As health care has offered longevity, today's 60s and beyond and up are the 40s and 50s of twenty years ago.

Four years back, at 70, during my 310-mile solo month and a half hike over the Superior Hiking Trail along Lake Superior – never one to believe in a hereafter – I thought:

'Wow.'

I realised, there had to be a higher force alerting me that if I were not more alert to danger, I would die. So, I got right to it and watched where I put my next step. At last, I now understood that I was not God or the centre of the Universe but a miniscule dot on its perimeter.

Socialisation is essential. There is no more fun for me – loads of other cross-country ski maniacs around me – than when the starting gun goes off. Except if the police are chasing me. As we exercise and just exult in being alive, we are all role models for each other or others.

It is hell to grow old but the alternative sucks. I want to grow older younger. It is crucial to stay vital. Hang out with young people. Do not retire unless you must. I can never comprehend why people count the days until retirement and, when they do so, dry up and blow away. More about that later. Make plans. Rediscover yourself but be mindful of realistic challenges as I lay them out. I am a notoriously lousy driver. I do not like driving and am not particularly good or safe at it. I will not drive a yellow bus at seven in the morning with wild and crazy tired (from texting their friends all night) teenagers. I will not deliver parts for Napa.

Growing older than 60 was always something that happened to someone else. The gray or no hair, the paunch (men spread out like apples, women like pears), was a giveaway. Now, I am 78. I am motivated by the fact that I refuse to act my age and would like to convey this life attitude. If I check out Sunday's obits, I do not check the ages of those unfortunate to have passed on. We have optimistic expectations for how long we will live. Actuarial tables based on my lifestyle and the parents I did not choose, I am likely to hit 94.

It is realistic to accept that we have limited earth time. Again, I accept that there is a mystical force – not saving me – but reminding me that if I'm not careful, I'm going to die sooner than scheduled. I comfort myself that I have predetermined my body will go to The University of Minnesota School of Medicine. I hope aspiring doctors do not giggle over my body as I did over Ethyl, my designated medical school cadaver. She did not look great after we were done. She did not look great when we started.

Men Over 60 is not a self-improvement book. My wish is that it be entertaining as well as enlightening. I want to explain feelings we all have about that final Uber ride to the great beyond. How can we accept what we do not know or understand? Rather than obsessing about where we go next, avoid negative thoughts, maximise health, and grow older younger.

As I did in my earlier book, addressing men's challenges at 40, I spice most chapters about men over 60 who although knowing the importance of acknowledging the grim reaper, must also move on. This book is meant to pick up where *Dr D's Handbook for Men Over 40* left off but with new concerns. This book is not about denial. It does not advise temperance, quitting, or neurosing. *Men Over 60: Do Not Quit Now!* offers solid advice about what to expect hurdling past 60, all the while accepting the next challenge of our lives, and not quitting despite the inevitable.

JAMA, the esteemed medical journal, reminds us that, "The number of persons older than 60 is expected to double from 2010 to 2050, increasing from 40.2 million to an estimated 88.5 million." Such statistics warn of the negative impact of an increasing elder population on the work force. What will be the cost to the health care system?

Fellow athlete, Roy Carlstad whom I profiled in *Dr D's Handbook*, was still out on the ski trail at 90 plus. An electrician, he had been retired for decades. Since last I wrote about Roy, he had lost his wife of many years to cancer and, unlike most men our ilk who are not equipped to cook or clean as their spouses once did for them, Roy thrives as a bachelor. Outwardly, he would say he was comfortable with his life but missed his wife. There are other downsides for a ninety plus despite he has stayed wonderfully active. His daughter confides he can be forgetful especially finding his way on a several hours drive north to their lake home.

Last time I skied with him; it was a sunny cold Minnesota winter day. It is 20 years since we had skied together on a backwoods trail. He has all the life and juice of a man 20 years his junior. Roy is an example of the benefits of a vigorous life. The guy's an Eveready battery. If he is not skiing, he is on his road bike. It is difficult to believe that Roy had a quadruple bypass 10 years back. Alas, Roy elected not to do ski marathons any longer.

A long-lost friend from my Dartmouth days, the esteemed Reverend Brewster "Budge" Gere, who has written the spirituality chapter for the book, quotes Ecclesiastes to help us enter this later chapter of our lives. His perspective about how important it is to find spiritual meaning over 60 convinced me to journey back for my 50th college reunion. That decision runs counter to why I had not returned since my 25th arrogantly claiming that I did not attend reunions because I did not want to be around old people.

We need not see ourselves as either conquerors or the vanquished. Cooperation, harmony, tranquillity, peacefulness, and serenity can become our new companions, filling our hearts with positive thoughts, freeing our minds to focus on important matters, saving our energy for living life fully, and appreciating each day as never before.

Chapter 1
Fear of Dying

I have pride that I have the strength that puts me in the top 1% of fitness in the over-70 set. Men *Over 60: Don't Quit Now!* can allay fear of dropping dead from a sudden infarct or a killing arrhythmia. This chapter explains why, with consistent exercise, our maximal heart rate drops, and why we should still screen for narrowed coronaries. Progressive decrease in muscle mass and strength starts in our 30s. Ageing men still have great endurance but at a slower pace. Marathoners who have done 100s of marathons can develop enlarged hearts, and, atrial fibrillation, accompanied by congestive heart failure. When the latter happens, cardiac output deteriorates when conduction circuits may become disrupted.

"Man cannot possess anything as long as he fears death. But to him who does not fear death, everything belongs. If there is no suffering, man would not know his limits, would not know himself."

– Leo Tolstoy

I suggest we refute ageism. Society wants to believe we should "Take it easy," or "Act your age." "There's no fool like an old fool." I encountered family hysteria as I embarked on my 310-mile mid-May through mid-to-late June solo "through" hike on The Superior Hiking Trail from Duluth, Minnesota to Canada. "Dad, come back, please come back," was how my eldest daughter reacted.

Key words for such an experience starting in northern Minnesota mid-May: cold, tough hills, mud, no sign of humanity, and horizontal rain. Mid-June brought mosquitos. I did not quit. I did not bail. I thought about quitting my trek constantly, especially when I was soaked through and near hypothermia. I realised before long that there was some mysterious force not about to save me but rather, to send me a message that if I kept being such a dumb shit I could die. More about that later.

Research shows that those of us over 60 think and fret about death and dying less than men in their 40s. Every day, as I brush my teeth, a look at the mirror reminds me I am not going to be the first man to score at the local bar. Even worse, as a Gray Panther, I find myself being called "Sir". Are we invisible or have we just become superfluous? Gone are Greek and Roman times when our opinion in the agora meant something.

Hey, here is a reality bite. Just check out Social Security statistics that proclaim, "A man reaching 65 today can expect to live, on the average, until 84." Also, the longer we live, the longer we live. One quarter of our ageing population will live beyond 90. One tenth will live past 95. The number of people over 60 will increase by 2050 and represent 8–10% of the total population. As a larger cohort, the number of the elderly will jump to 22% of the total population by 2050. Why won't I be there to party as well?

A question that sometimes disturbs me, "Do I want to live that long? How good will my life be at the top of the age pyramid?" I am not convinced I want to become a member of "The Frail Elderly". What does Woody Allen say?" I have nothing against death, I just don't want to be there."

I as well.

The questionnaire for My 50th Dartmouth reunion asked, "What would you do differently, if you could do it all over again?"

My answer, "I can't."

Appendix 1 will give you a fix on the criteria determining your life expectancy. A great deal has to do with the parents you did not choose. So much as well, is about lifestyle. Do you smoke? Do you use drugs? How many drinks do you have a week? How much stress is there in your life? How many hours do you sleep a night? What do you eat?

Am I in denial? I am all about delaying the reality that I will die. Michael Douglas, in *The Kominsky Method* says, living longer is about "Coming to grips with the reality of getting older… It is also about friendship. It's about what happens if your dreams don't come true and another dream comes up." Like many of my friends, I wrestle with my fear of death by denying it.

Judy Passfill warns, "The thing about growing old is that you have to accept it – if you don't, you'll be miserable as sin. You've got to try and find the few good things about it."

My medical classmate, retired orthopaedist, Dr Fred Buechel, realistically reminds me. "I have far less time in front of me than behind me."

As things were heading several years back, and I was not thinking pre-emptively and kept falling, I worried I would not reach 78. But who knows? When it is my time, I opt for a quick and peaceful death. French philosopher, palaeontologist, and Jesuit, Pierre Teilhard de Chardin, opined, "Growing old is like being penalised for a crime you haven't committed."

I may be in denial that I too am ageing fast by avoiding high school and college reunions. and why shouldn't I? I don't seem to have anything in common with contemporaries from college 50 years ago who just seem to have checked out of an active life. I see them in my alumni magazine standing around with a cocktail in one hand next to an equally ageing partner. I wonder if they have tickets for the next cruise ship to watch whales mating off the Kenai Peninsula. According to the late Billy Graham, "Growing old has been the biggest surprise of my life," I'm also insulted that some refer to those of us over 70 as "the very old". I do not want anyone to include me in that category!

Ed Koch, the once controversial multiple-term mayor of New York City, said, "It is a little disappointing to see your legs are not as strong. But I like the idea of growing old, and the thought of approaching death is not particularly daunting to me." I wish I were as sanguine as the late and controversial mayor of The Big Apple.

If I watch my friends becoming 80, I know there is an inevitable and more rapid decline over the next decade of my life. The statistics confirm this. Younger fellow athletes honour those seniors who persevere. Now, I am the surprised recipient of such esteem. At the biggest cross-country ski races in North America, the 55 or 28K American Birkebeiner, they have dedicated a special wave to those of us over 70. We can be easily identified by the "70" emblazoned on our special bibs. I proudly wear my logo of respect. At least, it is not a Depends Diaper.

Doctor "Art" Leon laughs describing how his daughter reacted when she saw him competing in his forties in a master's track event.

She asked, "How come all those other guys are running and you're walking?"

We cannot avoid ageing no matter how hard we try. With age, functions decline. Our bodies inevitably are losing certain sensory perceptions – how we interact with our environment – at variable rates. Motor activities – how we do things - decline. Cognitive performance – how we multitask or just remember something as simple as names or days and recent memory especially – may waver. Many admit they have a bit of the "Can't Remember shit Syndrome" (CRS). Personal and societal expectations should not influence how we believe our physical activity can endure with age.

At the start of another gonzo cross-country ski race last winter, all of us, decked out in lycra racing suits as thin as panty hose and feeling colder than hell, stood anxiously waiting for the starting gun.

"How old are you?" I ask the younger guy fidgeting at the starting line next to me.

"Thirty-two," he replies.

"You?" he asks.

"Oh, I'm 75."

I feel like a geriatric stud.

"I want to be like you when I'm your age."

He shoots back.

Envious, I answer, "I want to be like you at thirty."

We both laugh as the gun goes off.

There is still no greater thrill for me when the starting gun goes off... and I am not being chased by the police. In college I was.

He does not know what I know: two stents, two shoulders trashed, and an arthritic toe. My internist asks as he looks at the x-rays of my neck.

"What's with that T2 compression fracture?"

My answer.

"Oh, I think that may have happened when I did a 360° out in the woods skiing, or maybe it was when I hit a pothole at the bottom of a long hill biking to work."

There is a pause before the starting gun goes off. Then with a rush of adrenaline I am in a stampede, poles flying, a few racers screaming, "You're on my pole." "Comin' through." Uh, oh, someone was not careful. Snap. Now he has two poles for the price of one.

"I need a pole. I need a pole!" the guy next to me screams.

It is Sunday morning. I could be home sipping a latte, staring at my recovery poodle, and reading the Sunday paper. Oh, I think I got that decision backward.

I have a little secret. I really go to see my internist just to see how he is doing. Aside from my usual aches and pains, especially, from training hard that morning for the ski racing season, I have a smile on my face. My doctor admits he feels OK. I know I do.

There is no lying to a mirror. I see those wrinkles every time. A mirror tells no lies. My wrinkles are crevasses. As seniors, we take an exponential number of pills related to our age. I take eleven pills at night and four in the morning; that is, if I do not drop them into the toilet. I always had thought such a mishap was a myth until it happened to me... more than once.

How did 70 sneak up on me? Where did my competition go? Something happened at 70. Are my competition in nursing homes, dead, have gone south for the winter, or just cannot slip a Depends Diaper into their racing suits?

I am no longer skiing against 50 or 100 guys my age. I am lucky to see a field of 15 to 20. I still feel competitive. The alternative I entertained for only half of a minute was to turn in my racing suit, head out to California, trade in my Sorrels for flip flops, and long johns for worn khaki Bermuda's and an old t-shirt. Many over 60 decide to forgo the discipline required to continue training for racing. Or maybe, it is the pain they no longer can tolerate. Then, I quickly realise neither my daughters nor I could endure more than a week together.

The unwillingness to endure high end physical challenges turns plenty of elders away and toward the links. I go out and it is 20 below. My nostrils freeze. My nose did last winter-twice. The snow makes that crunchy sound when it is below 0 degrees. With age, it is extremely hard to keep my hands warm. It is mittens or pain. Whoever wrote "Life for many men over 60 is enormously fruitful and exciting," was written by someone younger than 70. But why can't it still be a great time of life?

Once over 60, we can delay unnecessary declining strength, agility, and flexibility. I love the quip, "I'm not getting older, I'm just getting slower." An extreme decline does not have to happen so fast. The decline – a reality bite – does not have to happen so uncontrollably or so severely. Staying active and vital can slow the inevitable. Accept realistic changes rather than flailing, struggling, or avoiding the truth. Stay physically and cognitively active!

We can continue to maintain independent living. Sometimes, we must convince our loved ones we still have the juice. We can continue enjoying a good quality of life. We must maintain a positive physical and mental relationship with our environment. Many belittle or minimise our capabilities. They are wrong.

A year ago, I realised I was falling more. After enough accidents, I realised I was making bad choices. I learned to anticipate, to think first, and act second. We must approach risky activities more carefully than when we were younger. I have NOT lost the ability to stay upright. I realised I needed to slow it down a bit. I am running out of my nine lives. I realise I must think before I act.

Recently, I took a painful tumble after I decided to climb up to a sweet look-out that looked out over miles of the Minnesota River valley. Everything went well until the journey back down. The tread on my boots had worn. I had failed to anticipate I needed shoes with better traction. There was glare ice under the slushy snow. Wham, down I went. Luckily, I did not break a hip or rib, but whacked some big muscles over the back of my pelvis. It took several painful months before it healed.

The worst accident was yet to come. I became distracted for a second talking with a friend as we went side-by-side on a downhill over boiler-plate manmade snow on our cross-country skis. I caught a ski tip and did a header. After driving myself to the ER with the worst headache of my life and stopping every mile to vomit, the ER doctor gave me the good and bad news. The good news was, "You didn't break your nose." The bad news was. "You have a subdural hematoma and you're going into the NICU." I spent a good part of the next week somewhere in the vicinity of Pluto as the doctors carefully lowered my blood pressure to stabilise my subdural bleed. They were able to: no burr holes.

The vital ingredients that ensure our safety as we soar past 60 and our balancing ability adjusts to age, is that we need good judgment how and where to exercise. Just as with driving – we must stay focused.

Worry less about dying and more about staying fit. Ignore stereotypes or hysterical warnings from those who would confine us to the "Lazy Boy". My daughter had ill-founded fears when she heard about my planned 310-mile solo trek over the Superior Hiking Trail along the North Shore of Lake Superior.

I made it. Sure, our youthful capabilities may be on the decline at about the same speed as our testosterone. There is no denying it. We can make ageing more tolerable by challenging our bodies. We should not ignore reality. Our body and mind devolve. We must strengthen and build muscle to avoid losing what we have got.

- It is physically and mentally important to exercise to a sweat for 30 minutes at least three maybe four times a week.
- Do resistance/strength workouts three or four times a week.

We are on the decline after 60. There is the issue of losing muscle mass. You may notice that your gluts are shrinking by how it has become harder to hold your pants up.

Adequate muscle mass can make the difference between dependency and autonomy. Sign me up for the latter. Get plenty of resistance exercise to continue building muscle. Refill your glycogen stores after vigorous prolonged exercise. Don't skimp on protein in your diet. Some fat is good too.

Just as I warned in *Dr D's Handbook*, I could drop dead at 60 just as easily as I might have at done at 40 doing another hard repeat on a hill, or bringing my pulse to my calculated maximal heart rate (220–78=142). A graduated stress test will only go to 85% of your max. What else could my doctor really find if I can do a 48 K ski marathon and not have symptoms of angina – radiating arm pain, chest discomfort, or increasing shortness of breath that comes and goes? Ergo, I do not need a stress test-a personal decision.

Dr Leon addresses the issue of dropping dead during high intensity exercising. His recommendation is that even men at a higher risk for coronary artery disease will benefit from "light and moderate non-work physical activity". Those who exercise at almost any level have lower rates of mortality than inactive men. Increasingly, exercise physiologists recommend interspersing bursts of speed, called High Intensity Interval Training (HIIT), into workouts. Jane Brody, our New York Times exercise savant, reports HIIT is even safe for those with heart or lung disease. The axiom is that if we train fast we race faster.

Do not surrender without a fight. Robert E. Lee did not at Appomattox. That is why I continue to train, coach, instruct, and to race cross-country skiing. Hang in there. If you have not already been exercising, get a good check-up periodically. That can include a resting cardiogram (EKG) – especially if you have risk factors such as diabetes or hypertension. It's not a bad idea, if you have acute or old changes on your EKG, to undergo a monitored graduated stress test (GXT).

Then get going! Start a realistic exercise program – not too hard, not too easy. If you are not sure how to accomplish this, get a trainer. The worst mistake can be to start out too hard, then hurt like hell, and end up quitting. As I mentioned *in Dr D's Handbook*, *if* your trainer is fantastic and single, marry her (him).

Look optimistically at ageing. If your age group on the racing circuit is shrinking, that gives you a better chance to jump onto the podium. When folks say, "Good luck," before a race, I tell them, 'It's not about luck. Longevity is about how long your mom or dad lived. Lifestyle habits also determine how long you will live. Go at it, lads!'

The challenge is to not stop. Do not quit but realistically be open to adjust your fitness goals. Two coronary stents saved my life two decades ago. Improved vision from two successful cataract surgeries several summers ago also changed my life and goals. Now, I can see white and blue again. A chronic rotator cuff has responded to overhead pulley exercises extending range of motion of my shoulder, stretching the capsule, and minimising pain. A left shoulder acromial-clavicular (AC) separation looks bad but does not limit my range of motion or elicit pain. Lifting five-and ten-pound hand weights and stretching with the girls in my barre class three times a week has strengthened both shoulders. No more injections. When I feel pain, rather than quitting, I work the shoulder exercises and I am back in action. Voila!

Thank you, higher spirit, that I am not yet frail. I watch my friend Dick, a retired doctor as well, but now over 80. He is shuffling, bent over, and no longer great in the balance and driving departments. Dick is older – not by much.

If I look back at my mother's ageing, I recollect her winning the 65-and-older singles tennis championship on Chris Evert's home court in Ft. Lauderdale.

But she died at 73 from childhood renal disease, metastatic breast cancer, and severe coronary complications. Some of successful ageing is genetic, but there is no escaping other illnesses affecting men over 60 that I describe in a later chapter.

A 50th College Reunion Challenge: A Change of Heart

Rev. Brewster "Budge" Gere, my college classmate, who has written the spirituality chapter, encouraged me to return for my 50th reunion. He knew that I needed closure and resolution. A retired minister and now, by default, our class chaplain, understood that I unconsciously wanted closure.

He tells us in the spirituality chapter of his passion to assist us to not fear ageing, but rather to savour the joy of wonderful memories when we were invincible – or so we thought. He knows how important our gathering would mean to those, like myself, who still savour life. At the memorial service at the reunion, he recited the names of those who had already passed. The process was one of letting go and saying goodbye. As he read their names, I cried. Afterward, I felt cleansed, at peace, and less fearful of my own inevitable death.

I knew I had made the right decision after I met a familiar aged guy on the bus on the last leg of my journey back to Hanover, New Hampshire for the reunion. He looked vaguely familiar despite the unavoidable age-changes of fifty years.

I leaned over and asked, "Are you going where I'm going to, to our fiftieth reunion?" His answer was, "I am Bob, Peter. Remember me?"

This was the first of several scrimmages I would have fighting back tears. I realised this initial reluctant journey was the opportunity to savour the memory of innocence and excitement. The process, sometimes wistful, sometimes sad, sometimes tearful, awakened me to the value of the work ahead for me that early summer weekend.

Erik Erikson describes Eight Stages of Man. In the seventh, between 40 and 64, we ask, "Can I make my life count?" By the Seventh Stage, over 65, we are now elder and, hopefully, wiser. This will be the time to judge our lives as one of integrity or one we may perceive as less so. If we believe we have made a favourable contribution, we feel contentment. If we believe that we have not, we may feel despair.

Dartmouth of my time was notorious for discovering the hangover. Many of us had many wild adventures. As a gray-haired elder, I am now face-to-face recalling invincibility but, now it is more about invisibility. "Budge" helped me realise that I needed closure over our earlier breakfast that had made me take the leap and attend our fiftieth.

"Of course, you should go," he said assertively.

Everyone had changed. Most I greeted still showed spirit, calmly looking out through the wrinkles of age and wisdom earned.

One of my old study buddies asked, 'Do you remember how we spent hours talking endlessly by the corner of The Green, after we closed the library?'

I flashed back to the beauty of a cold New Hampshire night where we talked as my nostrils frosted. I quickly recalled our former innocence and bonding.

He reminded me, "We didn't care that it was minus 20."

Ah, I thought, *age is wasted on the young."*

We made up for lost time on those party weekends of the early 60s. Little sleep and ten too many beers were punishing on Monday. What we learned had little to do with the classroom. Truth and beauty hid in last-minute all-nighters when we crammed, an antidote of too little sleep and not enough books the past semester. The bonding lay not in hours of soporific lectures, but a friend who could distil all we needed to know in the final 12 hours before the exam.

"I'm way over my head. I will not pass!" I had exclaimed.

I did.

At the reunion there were enough hearing aids and canes to raise the value of hearing aid stocks 20 points. Everest and Jennings wheelchairs would also have sold well. I could visualise a booth in the alumni tent for wheelchairs, hearing aids, Viagra, and walkers. I felt indescribable joy reconnecting with men I had not seen for 50 years. Fortunately, our name badges were printed in large letters for a quick visual

I woke up one day no longer in later life crisis. My God, I am 75. The realisation was devastating as I realised, I must prepare for the end. I sobbed unexpectedly while in my physician's office for my physical. My mortality flashed graphically before me. I have had some medical challenges that surfaced earlier in my life and, fortunately, have resolved: angina with stents, and the earlier described subdural hematoma after my fall skiing.

I know that what I have suffered with ageing is far less than most men my age. The stents have worked for over 14 years. My subdural hematoma resorbed. Memory issues that were the consequences of the subdural improved after a month of memory therapy. I may be running out of my allotted nine lives. Now, after the several close calls, I'm less fearful of dying.

Like-minded men my age should question – even become militant – opposing common stereotypes society has about those of us who are over 60. Today's 70 is yesterday's 50. If given the opportunity and the wherewithal, any divorced or widowed septuagenarian can and could run off to Tahiti with Greta, the 54-year-old divorcee, pumping iron on the adjacent elliptical. Life is all about dispelling stereotypes.

If your body is willing and an enlightened internist approves, heed Jane Brody's advice. You still can run hard and fast. Get out there and challenge your body rather than schmoosing with your friend Phil about your failing body parts while walking around the lake. Recent studies purport such high intensity interval training (HIIT) mixed with your regular three-times a week workout is as safe as your regular moderate aerobic activities and can increase your speed. Sure, you are over 60. Take a risk. Yes, death is inevitable. Refuse to heed societal misconceptions about our physical and emotional abilities.

Spurts of maximum effort (HIIT) is safe even for someone with atrial fibrillation, controlled moderate heart failure, or COPD. It is all about tolerating pain. So much for aerobic cribbage or controlled pool floating. Pushing yourself to the max has its risks; sudden death from an arrhythmia or infarct; a fall, a ripped tendon or ligament; or sore muscles. I don't know about you, but I certainly are going to take the risk.

It is vital to prepare for new challenges. Assessing legitimate limitations such as with balance, gait, or strength is especially important. Aerobic activity, strength, and balance training can ward off muscle atrophy and unnecessary falls. It is crucial to think ahead to cognitively avoid going to ground. Be circumspect but, do not let inhibiting cultural stereotypes about what men over 60 can accomplish physically influence you. Don't let anyone rain on your parade. Realistically, question exaggerated societal fears of an older man dying suddenly, and instead, continue to gather the benefits of maintaining your body and mind.

Chapter 2
Physical Changes of Men Over 60

This chapter is the reality bite about physically ageing after 60. Apoptosis, programmed cell death, adversely affects cells. We lose over 30% of our muscle mass over our lifetime. Slow twitch fibres that favour endurance replace fast twitch fibres for speed. Posture is compromised. The chance of falling increases.

Restart and continue strength training and aerobic activities. Throw in bursts of speed. Add some plyometrics. Practice balance exercises. Men are apples, women are pears. Watch your waistline. Be mindful and proactive with your lipids especially total cholesterol, HDL, LDL, and triglycerides.

> "Those who think they have no time for bodily exercise will sooner or later find time for illness."
>
> – Edward Stanley (1826–1907)

What we want to do is maintain as best we can. We are talking preventing loss of muscle mass as best we can. There is that buzz word, sarcopenia. This is all about losing muscle mass that can accompany loss of joint flexibility. Looking at the average ageing male, we are going to lose 10–40% of our muscle mass every decade after 50. Muscle strength goes hand in hand with muscle mass. Concurrently, we also lose 12–14% muscle strength per decade. Why shouldn't you or I be the outlier?

We can develop a lifestyle that can reverse this trend or, at least, delay the inevitable. This way, we can feel equanimity toward the unavoidable reality of ageing and dying by pushing ourselves harder despite that our exercise upper limits declines. Statistics tell us that there is a drop in aerobic capacity of 30% over 50. Maximal oxygen uptake subsequently declines 0.5–1% a year. Those who insist on defying stereotypes must still face age-related limitations. Face them. Don't run from them.

Statistics define what is the norm or the average capability of what we can or cannot do: how fast we can run and jump, or, simply put, how strong we still are. We need to face and stabilise yet never can reverse changes in muscle strength, balance, and flexibility. Later chapters will give you the how-to; that is, how to maximise balance and gait to maintain these modalities. There are 35–40% more falls in in those of us over 60. At 78, I am concerned – even as a committed athlete – of an increasing number of falls I have had and offer advice how you can avoid them.

I love Doctor Leon's quote paraphrased from Hippocrates. "Parts of the body used in moderation… become thereby healthy, well developed and age more slowly…" I explained in *Dr D's Handbook for Men Over 40* the advantages versus the disadvantages of various levels of exercise. Is a marathon runner better protected from death more than a couch potato?

A Harvard study in the *American Journal of Cardiology* on the *Knee-Heart Connection*, discusses the connection" between ACL repair among former professional football players and later cardiovascular risk. There are more than 100,000 ACL repairs yearly. Those undergoing ACL repair during their professional football career had a 50% higher chance of a heart attack later in life.

Does exercising more and harder help you live longer? Exercise physiologists reassure us that more vigorous exercise does not offer additional protection from heart disease than moderate-intensity activities.

A kinesiologist, Dr Arthur Leon, explains that a moderate amount of predominantly light to moderate non-work exercise can reduce cardiac morbidity and mortality. As I explained in *Dr D's Handbook*, over-the-top exercisers – especially in the 40 and over set, have a higher incidence of sudden death from a fatal arrhythmia even if very fit. Men over 60, after a long history of endurance sport can develop left ventricular hypertrophy that can interfere with atrial circuitry leading to atrial arrhythmias. Atrial fibrillation, subsequently, can be the cause of heart failure due to compromised cardiac output. However, the good news is that there is not the same risk of sudden death as among the forties set.

We can certainly reduce risk factors by stopping smoking; reducing your waistline to less than 40 inches, decreasing your total cholesterol, upping your HDL lipids, lowering your LDLs, your "bad" cholesterol, losing weight, and lowering an elevated blood pressure. Another concern about the advantages or risks of a lifelong endurance exercise regimen, particularly noted among marathoners who have done hundreds of races, is an onset of cardiac rhythm disturbances, particularly atrial fibrillation (AF). Such long-term endurance athletes develop documented post-race elevated troponin levels consistent with heart muscle injury. Paradoxically, they also have structural changes to cardiac muscle including coronary artery plaques usually found in obese deconditioned individuals.

Dr Jostein Grimso of the Feiring Heart Clinic in Norway, in his longitudinal, 28 to 30-year follow-up study of long-term endurance cross country skiers, found a high prevalence of atrial fibrillation (AF) – European Journal of Cardiovascular Prevention and Rehabilitation, 17 (1) 2010.

He followed racers in the 54 km. Norwegian Birkebeiner Rennet from Rena to Lillehammer, Norway. A racers carries a 3.5 Kg back-pack-(the weight of the mythic king's son and heir to the Norwegian throne.) – commemorating his rescue in the 13th century in the Norwegian Birkebeiner (Birch Leggings) cross country ski race. This gruelling cross-country ski race crosses two mountains and elite athletes average over 15 mph over the flat sections of the course and up to 40 mph on some hills.

Grimso found that enlargement of the heart's left atrium – along with bradycardia (a pulse less than 60)appeared to be an important risk factor for AF among such long-term, endurance cross-country skiers.

'This atrial enlargement,' he said, "is the heart's adaptation to endurance training."

Thirteen of the 78 skiers studied (16.7%), experienced AF at some time during the 28–30 years of follow-up, with a current prevalence of 12.8%.

Professor Josep Brugada of the European Heart Rhythm Association (EHRA) in Barcelona describes the impact of AF as enormous: 5% of European medical expenditures are related to atrial fibrillation, and the most common rhythm disorder. Those of us who have exercised long and hard over the decades, have cardiac enlargement, AF, or heart failure, certainly significant enough to end a competitive career.

As I explained in *Dr D's Handbook* about cardiac risks for men over 40, such an issue of sudden death during strenuous exercise is certainly a possibility for those of us over 60. In the younger athlete, S. Chugh and J.B Weiss (*J Am College of Cardiology*, 2015) describe sudden death related to strenuous exercise may be related to cardiac enlargement – left ventricular hypertrophy (LVH) and described as an "athletic heart".

Peter McCullough, M.D., M.P.H, a cardiologist at Baylor University Medical Center in Dallas, calls such an enlargement the "athletic heart". He reports that in the younger athlete in their 20s and 30s, the most common cause of sudden death is hypertrophic obstructive cardiomyopathy. Researchers note otherwise among older long-term marathoners who have completed hundreds of marathons, that they experience heart muscle changes and the development of an abnormal circular heart rhythm, most often atrial fibrillation.

Robert Schwartz of the Minnesota Heart Institute using coronary CAT scans, notes increased coronary calcification (plaques) among long-term marathon runners, with an increased possibility of sudden death. Such athletes demonstrate cardiac enlargement and bradycardia. The clinical question is whether this is related to inflammation and scarring of heart muscle?

Schwartz notes that atrial fibrillation is epidemic among over-distance, long-term endurance athletes. Deteriorating race performance accompanies atrial fibrillation. Decreased cardiac output, ejection fraction, and athletic performance may ultimately lead to congestive heart failure unless the rhythm disturbance is corrected. I have seen one too many saddened marathon skiers or runners who, despite dedicated training, become dejected by the consequences of losing the long endurance sports they have loved. They then must adapt and enjoy life in the slow lane.

Researcher, James O'keefe at Mayo endorses regular exercise. Yet, they also have seen a correlation between chronic endurance training, excessive sustained exercise, and repetitive injury to cardiac muscle associated with heart failure. Carl Lavie in his 2015 study, concludes, "The overall benefits of running far outweigh the risk for most individuals and are associated with considerable protection against chronic diseases."

A progressive reduction in muscle mass and function starts back in our thirties to fifties and goes down, down, down from there. Muscle loss morphs in stages from presarcopenia to worsening sarcopenia, eventually contributing to "the fragility syndrome". That is why, rather than winning the overall race, we should accept that we now compete in five-year age categories and win!. Masters' competition starts at age 30 and rewards those who still value competition that requires dedicated training. We are all in this battle together. Loss of muscle mass occurs despite good intentions. Strength, especially in the lower extremities, decreases yearly. Here it is again; aerobic activity and strength training can stabilise albeit we now must adapt to winning our age group.

An older friend stoops forward as if he were watching each step. Senile posture is an unconscious forward tilt of our head as we age. Awareness of this change, concentration on your drooping head, may help avoid further tilt. (see Appendix 5) Hey, wait a minute, we ARE doing the best not just getting around, but keeping the spring in our step. Maybe, such an "old look", comes from checking out the path ahead of us so as not to go to ground. Just look at almost the same posture developing prematurely in the younger set, the consequence of constant texting.

If we stop exercising and strength training, from age 30 to 50, expect that muscle mass and strength will decline 1% a year. "Things get worse by 70," reports Doctor Leon. He notes, "The rate of loss jumps 3% a year." Over our lifetime, we can expect a 30% loss of muscle mass. We may experience a loss of posture, strength, and balance. Maintaining muscle strength is crucial.

Not always does it make sense to blame our parents. Dad just hated jogging, biking, and preferred bowling, and golf. No wonder, poor pops dropped on the 10th hole: the result of at a steak and golf diet. My mother past 65, had her first bout of angina playing a hard game of tennis doubles down at the park. Despite that she was a lifelong athlete, renal failure attributable to pyelonephritis as a child, subsequent coronary heart disease(CHD), and, finally, metastatic breast cancer. She died peacefully at 73. She just said, "Peter, I am stopping dialysis."

I had my angina, two blocked coronaries, and life-saving stents after my world imploded around 62 with losses of the worst kind. I believe in the mind-body connection. No wonder people talk about dying of a broken heart. Stress, stress, and more stress. That is all about sustaining a job, a nasty boss, wrinkles in our marriage, or difficult adult children.

In our forties, our greatest risk was thinking we were invincible. As we soar into and over the landmark 60s, the challenge is now about rationalising if we have made our mark on society.

A few summers back, I fulfilled another fantasy from my bucket list, rehabbing a '65-foot Chris Craft Roamer at the end of the Bayfield, Wisconsin city dock on Lake Superior, while enjoying the beauty of the Apostle Islands. On my breaks, I sat on the foredeck, coffee cup in hand, watching the line of Wisconsin tourists waiting to board the tour boat on the next mooring from our boat. Most of the vacationers appeared overweight. My observation confirms the statistics that being overweight or obese is the major American epidemic of the

21st century. Ours is the Land of Plenty; too much food, too little exercise other than hefting a craft beer from table to our mouth. Perhaps, my observations do seem to confirm that Wisconsin is indeed, the cheese and beer capital of the US.

Like it or not, in the not-so-distant future, I will most likely need someone at my elbow as I negotiate a walker or push forward in my wheelchair. As I was growing up, my father was confined to a wheelchair from the polio he contracted in 1949. He was the sole survivor in his hospital ward, and after nine months in an iron lung and another half year rehabilitating (as did FDR) at Warm Springs, Georgia, he built and became an awesome administrator of a modest rehabilitation centre specialising in head and neck trauma.

When my sartorially dressed father visited each new patient, he was inspiring as he demonstrated that their new life still had value. For thirty years he had a wonderful cartoon on his office wall of two nurses whispering to each other as a demonic appearing patient in his wheelchair appeared at the ready, hands on his wheels.

"Watch out for Mr Jones, he just had his wheels oiled." Too bad my dad had chain smoked his entire life. He succumbed to metastatic lung cancer at age 65.

I visit my doctors periodically to see if they are OK. I am in better shape at 78 than my internist at 55. His nurse takes a double take when she sees my pulse is less than 40." She wonders aloud, "Is he in heart block"
'No.'

My doctor laughs.

"He does marathons."

Another example of challenging misconceptions about ageing. At a recent master's championship in Minneapolis, the largest contingent of competitors was in the over 60 set. You could not guess their age when you watched them registering.

Men over 60 have an age-related drop in the number of fast-twitch muscle fibres. Physiological cell death is called apoptosis... also described as cell suicide; that; programmed cell death. This is when more cells die than regenerate. We can lose the ability to build the antioxidants that fight harmful free radicals. Being overweight may affect our endocrine system demonstrated by adult-onset diabetes-when insulin loses the ability to properly metabolise glucose. More about that in the chapter about medical illnesses in men over 60.

We should return to the mantra that is the basis of *Men Over 60*. Leon advises, "Don't forget resistance training." Try sit-ups, push-ups, pull-ups, ideally, three or four times a week. If you are bored, try ear buds, watching the news as you peddle, and, especially, maintain a realistic but consistent schedule."

He advises 30 to 60 minutes of continuous aerobic exercise (Moderate to vigorous). Try fast walking or running. Better to jog than sit. Try upping the pace so you get up a light sweat. Develop flexibility by stretching. Stretch the major muscle groups: your calves, hamstrings, "quads", strong back muscles, triceps, and biceps, before and after exercise. FYI: If I develop a pain while running, I will stop and stretch again. It works.

When I am at the gym, in addition to a half-hour sweating on the elliptical and a circuit of three reps of 10 on the machines, I like to do some squats on a Bosu Ball to mix resistance and balance. I tell my friends who ask why I like the Bosu Ball. I tell my younger partner, Nada, that I do so because I am auditioning for Cirque du Soleil. I am the envy of the geriatric set. Some have tried, few have succeeded.

A regular exercise plan works. Believe the researchers who have studied the beneficial effects of all types of exercise. Exercise helps the younger set. So too, those of us over 60 will benefit immeasurably against the vortex of ageing by adhering to disciplined (but fun!) exercise. By exercising, we may be able to subdue accelerated cell death. We can mobilise our own antioxidants. that manage inflammation leading to cell destruction

I admire an eighty-year-old woman who joins me at barre class several times a week. She realises exercise maintains her mobility and is good for her head. She modifies the moves to fit her abilities—not age!

I do not expect to be another Charles Atlas, and certainly not another Richard Simmons. Maintaining muscle strength works for me and can, as well, for the so-called "frail" elderly. By doing as, I am hoping to delay my own progression to the inevitable.

I attribute recent and repetitive falls to bad judgment by not anticipating potential danger. I attribute most of my falls to bad decisions I made where I hike or run. I am increasingly more aware before I take my next step off a curb.

With long slow distance exercise, capillaries in lower extremities proliferate and makes exercise more efficient so muscles more efficiently oxygenate and improve cardiac output.

Losing or gaining weight each have their cheerleaders. I eat all the time to keep my weight stable. I pack it away. However, older men eat less. Taste buds atrophy like everything else in our bodies and we may have less motivation to eat. *Under the Spreading Atrophy*, was SJ Pearlman's quintessential humourist's take on ageing.

Diet among those over 60 impacts on exercise. A "Tea and Toast" diet-especially among widowed men - those who are divorced later in life. Decline in nutrition among the elderly may have dire consequences such as anaemia, accelerated muscle wasting, vitamin deficiency, and even unanticipated cognitive decline. Not eating right is detrimental. Eating right is crucial. That is how we can maintain muscle and a myriad of life's essential functions.

All the food groups are vital. Carbohydrates replenish the glycogen stores in muscle and the liver, and are vital for endurance activities. Cognitive clarity in the brain is dependent on glucose to sustain brain function. Proteins build muscle. Fats are vital components to fabricate hormones, teaming up with proteins for important neurological structures such as nerve sheaths. In the nutrition chapter, I will explain how eating patterns compliment an exercise plan. Do not quit now. Keep at it. Slow down the inevitable. Exercise and eat right. But of all else be happy as you do it. Make exercising fun.

Chapter 3
Cognition and Brain Function

"You should pray for a healthy mind in a healthy body."
    –   Juvenal, Satirist and Poet Second Century, AD

The relative severity of ageing-associated cognitive changes – how the brain functions – is clinically classified into three major categories, (1) Primary age-associated memory impairment (AAMI); (2) Mild cognitive impairment (MCI); and (3) Dementia. The progression ranges from AAMI, "benign forgetfulness", with some brain changes, to MCI, a compromised ability to perform routine activities of daily living (ADLs); and (3) Dementia, with inflammatory brain processes associated with an inability to perform most to all routine daily activities.

The four categories of cognition are speed, visuospatial, control, and executive. The prevalence of reported dementia in the U.S.A over 75 is approximately 5.2 million with 400,000 new cases- 25% over 75, and 40% over 80, due to Alzheimer's – plaques and tangles, or vascular damage from many small strokes.

Someone with unexplained forgetfulness, moodiness, and a decline in everyday activities can go down a torturous path of self-deception and denial. Someone can admit, "Oh, hell, I go upstairs and forget why I went up there in the first place." However, someone with dementia may begin to forget people, places, and things they knew well. He can become disoriented after shopping at Walmart. He asks, "Where did I park my car?" I have the ugliest and most visible color car color. I can always find it in a parking lot.

Keep exercising! This is one way to fight an absence of purpose in one's life, or the loss of friends or family. Depressed? Find out why. Resist a temptation to curl up and die after retirement. Avoid dropping out. Do not quit an active lifestyle and succumb to what the French call ennui, the act of not acting. Exercise improves mood, the negativism of depression, and enhances self-esteem.

Cognitive clarity may deteriorate from an array of mental disorders. The struggle with depression, anxiety, and bipolar disorder may affect cognition. Overwhelming grief, injury, or sickness can cloud the thinking process. Loved ones often do not understand why someone in their lives has become distracted, flighty, tangential, or inattentive.

Someone with bipolar disorder can demonstrate subtle or profound impaired thinking and judgment. Frederick Goodman and Kay Redfield Jamison in *Manic Depressive Illness: Bipolar Disorders and Recurrent Depression,* describe lapses in memory function with bipolar disorder that includes sensory, short and long-term memory, unconscious motor skills, and planning lapses.

Specifically, categories of brain function include long and short-term memory, association, comparison, verbal and quantitative abstract reasoning, spatial ability, manipulation, and synthesis.

Society unfortunately, does not tolerate unacceptable behaviour even when someone is depressed or an addict. My message, "Don't scare the horses in the street." Whatever the cause, as our brain devolves, executive control that plans actions and coordinates brain functions controlling appropriate behaviour may become painfully absent.

Pseudodementia can be how depression presents in older men and women over 60. Depression in an elderly family member can also masquerade as psychosis, confusion, memory loss, forgetfulness, an inability to focus, or disorientation. Quick mental status questions are, "Who is the president? What month or day of the week is it? Where are we? What am I showing you, Remember several numbers, or Identifying the time of day on a clock?"

For those close to the errant person, why performance or interactive behaviour deteriorates is of less importance than its consequences. Wild brain circuitry of mood disorders like depression, anxiety, or bipolar disorder may play havoc with executive function, affect energy, memory, processing speed, as well as psychomotor abilities.

Brain circuitry can become chaotic and affect global memory. Cognitive testing reflects Leonard Cohen's tale of woe, "I can't remember what, I can't remember when, I can't remember where."

School and work performance can deteriorate into a vortex of negative consequences. Lapses of executive function can lead to bad choices affecting profession and family.

Acute head trauma for someone over 60 from repetitive concussions, an intracerebral bleed, a traumatic subdural or epidural hematoma can lead to early dementia. A man over 60 with a history of traumatic brain injury (TBI) may struggle remembering names, numbers in sequence, or orientation.

Anecdotal reports suggest that with higher levels of physical and mental activity, memory gets a boost. After a TBI, occupational therapy can provide techniques for remembering names, numbers in sequence, and other memory patterns. I know it did for me after my subdural hematoma after my bad fall skiing.

Dr Leon explains that physical activity, especially aerobic exercise of sufficient intensity and volume, enhances cognitive performance that he calls the "Polypill". Leon emphasises that "even modest exercise attenuates the effects of brain ageing associated with cognitive decline, reduces major health problems, and lowers the risk of all-cause dementia."

Establishing a pattern of consistent and tolerable aerobic exercise of a level that works for you, can be your "Polypill", and keep you in your mental game. In 2011, Eric Ahlskog reported that middle-aged and older individuals who regularly exercise, experience less mental fall away and less risk for developing cognitive decline or all-cause dementia later.

Summon up motivation. Decide on a plan and how intensely you want to exercise. Develop a personal work-out schedule or have a professional trainer help you make one. Staying physically fit rather than living a sedentary lifestyle maintains brain health.

Multi-tasking presents challenges even among those who are highly disciplined. Older professional musicians explain that they must practice longer. A bassoonist with the St. Paul Chamber Orchestra opines, "We just cannot spontaneously concertise like our younger colleagues. We need to practice for concerts more than we did earlier in our careers."

Decision making is also vital. An example of compromised thinking is a man in his 70s or 80s mistakenly climbing trees, cleaning gutters two stories up but forgetting to secure and position the ladder correctly. Maybe, have your wife stand on the bottom rung. Set up the ladder correctly. Know when and where not to climb.

There are just too many stories about bad decisions – cognitive again – to climb onto the roof or to prune an apple tree ten feet up, culminating in a fatal fall. The fall often has nothing to do with balance but more to do with anticipating potential danger. The logical question is what was a man in his 70s or 80s doing up there in the first place?

Studies of both younger and older individuals who exercise regularly demonstrate faster reaction times and processing speed than those who are sedentary. In case you care, rats running on an exercise wheel react faster than sedentary rats.

Executive control initiates from the prefrontal and frontal lobes, the location where cognition begins to deteriorate earliest. Exercise improves oxygen to these and other important parts of the brain. Aerobic activities significantly maintain all brain functions, especially cognition. It affects how effectively we process information, how we continue to maintain executive function, and how we continue to make effective decisions.

In summary, aerobic activities can play an important role in decreasing depression, anxiety, cognitive decline, and, worst yet, dementia. Exercise also can increase self-efficacy and self-esteem.

So, take the "Polypill". Think right and let the games begin. *Mens sana in corpore sano*, a sound mind in a sound body.

Chapter 4
Balance, Posture and Locomotion

As we enter and pass our sixties, we must deal with increased vulnerability. We must adjust our activities by coping constructively with decreasing muscle mass and strength. Compromised balance can lead to falls, hip fractures, and loss of independence. Cataracts, macular degeneration, compromised proprioception – a malfunctioning vestibular system-are the culprits. It is not unusual that a man or woman of any age to experience sudden dizziness. This sudden disabling situation known as benign paroxysmal positional vertigo (BPPV) indicates our internal gyroscope has gone haywire, when the little stones and hairs in our semi-circular canals have gone haywire. We must cognitively anticipate a grandson's fire truck, or black ice. There it is again, Think first, act second

"The most important thing is posture: when you get old, it's the way you walk, the way you stand, that shows it."
— Carine Roitfeld, author

How we function and feel derives from how our body works. Balance, posture, and locomotion are essential to our relationship with gravity. Preferring unadorned classical music, I confess I do not know a pirouette from an arabesque. Unwittingly, I have demonstrated one or the other in plenty of falls. According to the Centers for Disease Control and Prevention, one-fourth of Americans older than 65 fall each year. Plus, every 11 seconds, an older adult is treated in the emergency room for a fall. Tragically, an older adult dies from a fall every 19 minutes.

Falls in our age set are caused by muscle weakness, impaired balance, a gait problem, environmental hazards, misusing prescribed medications; but primarily, in my not-so-humble opinion, the failure to anticipate danger. Of late, I do not fall as often since I accepted, I cannot reverse my age to 47 rather than 78. We also fail to anticipate potential hazards. One such unanticipated challenge can be stepping on a throw rug on a slick wooden floor on the way to the bathroom at four in the morning.

All was well until my fall in front of my cross-country -high school ski team at a freezing pre-practice meeting. I slipped, went to ground, tried to get up, but fell backwards twice. The team was kind to me. No one laughed, not even a snicker. After all, I was their pet old person. After that second attempt to stand up failed, I just lay there until the meeting ended.

I recall a similar embarrassing moment in my senior Dartmouth classics seminar. In a particularly dull moment, my classics professor had his legs

39

propped up at the head of the table. He quietly read from a worn copy of Catullus neatly propped on his lap, and waxing on-and-on, when he suddenly disappeared as he went backwards, only his argyles and Penny loafers visible at the end of the seminar table. Just as when I had fallen, no one laughed.

Another heavy hitter during a marathon-length race in the geriatric survivor category, just out of sight of the finish ahead of me, reportedly became dizzy and dropped. I only heard about his misfortune shortly after crossing the finish line only seconds behind him. He had already been carted off with hypothermia to the emergency tent.

A similar medical emergency befell another older competitor I had "duelled" with during another gruelling marathon. I did not see him at the finish line. I later learned that he passed out there and was whisked off to the ER with hypothermia and frostbite barely a minute in front of me. "Gray Panther down"! It is perverse, but why don't these guys self-destruct before the finish line? A thirst for competition is a demon despite our age.

With ageing, balance and mobility can slide insipidly downhill. Deconditioning or frailty can play an important role in our vulnerability. Many falls among those over 60 go unreported. We may hide an unwanted fall because evidence of instability and falling, if reported, could threaten our independence. When those who know and love us or a health care provider fear for our safety and fear we may be of danger to ourselves or to others, at least in Minnesota, they are required by law to report it.

In Abraham Maslow's hierarchy of needs about human behaviour, he explains that, to achieve self-actualisation and self-esteem, we must attend to our safety and physiological needs – far lower down the ladder of needs—first.

In mid-May, several years ago in my early 70s, I embarked on a 310 mile "through" hike on the Superior Hiking Trail from Duluth, Minnesota to the Pidgeon River, just over the Canadian border Canada. I made the mistake of telling my oldest daughter, Bria beforehand. She became hysterical.

'Daddy, Daddy, don't go, don't go!'

A discerning friend quipped, 'You'll never make more than a night.'

Obstinate to the core, I fooled both.

I did make it but, not without several near-death encounters. I am ageing in front of my children and, apparently, friends. Sometimes, when bad things happen, I realise they may be more realistic than I. As I will share later, I made it. But, with a few bumps on the rail. Would I move on to a longer trail like the Appalachian (AT) or the Pacific Crest Trail (PCT) No! Too little time left in my life to spend half a year hiking either on the AT or the PCT. I proved I could do it or shall I say endure it; that is, cold rain, mud, tough ups, and downs over boiling streams. But, the utter silence and the whole challenge, brought me back into myself.

I do not want to develop the senile posture prevalent among many of my peers. This is a posture many of the elderly develop. Senile posture is when our head and upper back begin to slowly bend forward. Are we assuming this position because we want to avoid falling over obstacles?

As our balance changes, failing to anticipate obstacles – grandkids' toys, throw rugs, the last step to the basement, or a curb on a walk can be our downfall. We forget we are no longer 30 and are more susceptible to falls. Loss of visual cues and an inability to anticipate or see upcoming objects are a major cause for a fall, when the chance of a fall increases. Appendix 4 provides exercises like chin tucks, wall tilts, wall arm circles, scapular retractions, and bird dogs that can help avoid senile posture.

Three important systems; vision, somatosensory, proprioception, and vestibular integrity determine good balance. I think of myself as an atypical late 70s guy because I regularly run, swim, hike, and bike. However, for older athletes, these and other exciting endeavours can be challenged by age-related negative effects of balance or coordination. In my case, I learned the hard way that I had to anticipate beforehand potential risks.

Two years ago I hurtled backwards from a four-foot shelf at work. I decided to shimmy up onto a shelf five feet from the floor. I rationalised I was a mountain climber in college. No sweats. My foot went through a board I was standing on and I went backwards. My agility and coordination allowed me to pull my leg up and out as I was falling backward. As I fell, I knew I was going to hit the floor and there was no way I could prevent it.

The back of my head hit, then bouncing off the concrete. There was a flash of light, and I had a second or two of nothingness. I am unclear why I was not severely injured. Luckily, the strong back muscles I have developed from cross-country skiing absorbed a great deal of the fall. I got up quickly but was shaky. I was afraid that if I told the manager exactly how I had fallen, I might lose my job for an illegal climb up to a platform without using a ladder. Fortunately, there were no witnesses. I gave an adulterated version of the fall to my manager. More than a little shaky, I biked home.

My back muscles that had taken the brunt of my fall hurt like hell for weeks. Fortunately, I did not have any symptoms of a concussion. I attribute my good fortune to some higher power not saving me, but telling me that if I keep being so dumb, I could die. Later that same winter, I became distracted on an easy downhill cross-country skiing, I caught a ski tip, and did a head and face plant on boiler plate hard, man-made snow. I went down too fast to throw my arms out. After cleaning up my face that had the appearance of a raw hamburger, I drove home, and suddenly developed a severe headache. Then I began projectile vomiting. My drive to the emergency room was harrowing. I had to pull over several times to vomit.

Once there, I was sent immediately for an emergency CAT scan of my head.

After the scan, the emergency room doctor came to my gurney and said, "I have good news for you. You did not break your nose. Now, the bad news – you have a sizeable subdural hematoma. I am admitting you to the NICU."

The neurosurgeon immediately ordered IV meds to lower my blood pressure. I cannot say I remember the next three days. Several days later, after some major confusion, the hematoma stabilised, and I escaped burr holes. If the pressure around my brain had escalated, it could have pushed it into the brain stem. I was fortunate. Serial CAT scans began to show the bleed had stopped, and over the next month, subsequent Cat scans showed the blood had resorbed.

"You were very close to getting burr holes," the physician assistant explained.

Several months later and after a month of memory rehab, I progressed from compromised memory to improvement by learning a new mnemonic, "SCARP", short, for Story, Categorisation, Association, or Pictures to more effectively remember someone I had just met or know, numbers, or things I was shown in sequence. The truth is I was never certainly not a Mensa candidate before or after the fall. During occupational therapy, I also learned my challenge has always been my distractibility and impulsivity.

My accident taught me that I cannot become distracted when I am engaged in active sports. Avoiding injuries of balance and gait are often cognitive. They often occur when we make bad decisions by acting before we consider risks. We may think our reaction times and balance are that of a man 20 years our junior. The reality is that balance inexorably changes when we are over 60.

After another fall moving fast and without anticipating the risk, I fell again on ice in the driveway, I was fearful the fall caused another bleed. The CAT scan did initially show some accumulating blood extending from the side of my brain toward the frontal lobe, the latter the centre for judgment, mood, and executive function. I was once again fortunate. The bleeding stopped. A CAT scan several weeks later showed no brain shift and the blood around my brain was resolving.

I experienced several more falls on the ice that winter. Doctors are the worst patients. I did a 42K marathon a few weeks after my subdural. I was careful not to fall. I wrongly denied I would fall, hit my head, or that I could extend the bleed. My decision was a risky one. I did have two more slips on the ice when I did not follow my own advice to think first, and act second, but, especially, to anticipate a possible mishap beforehand.

A light snowfall on black ice can be a prescription for disaster. Another run down the stairs and I fell backwards but broke the fall with my arm. I did not hit my head but could feel my brain going backward then forward. I worried my luck might be running out. I did not whack my elbow bad enough to break it. I did not dislocate my shoulder. I did not break my wrist or hip. These are all too frequently the casualties from a fall.

Several weeks later, I had another fall – an uncontrollable slide while walking my dog down a trail covered with soft snow and wearing boots with worn out soles. I fell backwards but rather than hitting my head, breaking a hip, my ribs, or spine, I smacked the big muscles at the back of my pelvis against a timber. I do not recall feeling pain like what I felt over the following weeks.

Inadvisably forgetting I am a senior, and walking too fast in flip flops heading for the steps down to the basement, I was suddenly in free fall, and I became airborne. I grabbed the heavy-duty curtains along the wall hoping to break my fall. I rolled as the floor, and I became one. No matter how agile I think I am, I know I need to anticipate danger.

The next refreeze day, on my daily walk with my trusty poodle, Saidie, I quickly jumped from my front step. With the sprint of a 30-year-old but the balance and gait of a septuagenarian, I did not anticipate the rain had made the step as slippery as a skating rink after the last turn of a Zamboni on a hockey rink. I lost control. I did the splits. I lucked out again this time, no visit to the ER. Clearly, accidents like these in men over 60 can be recurring. They can be prevented. I know I must anticipate and chart a safer course. I have had no more falls. How many lives have I used up?

I know now more than ever that I must take precautions when I change position. I now anticipate that black ice hides under a new layer of fluffy fresh snow from the night before. I learned the hard way the risk of skate skiing on the berm over slick ice on the lake. I went down again, but, this time, missed another brain shift.

Falls occur in 60% of men over 60 and are most often errors of judgment. Repeated head trauma contributes with ageing to cognitive decline. There can be serious long-term consequences of traumatic brain injury. Dr Leon reports, "A period of unconsciousness with a traumatic brain injury (TBI), especially with prolonged loss of consciousness of 30 minutes or more-at any stage of life-is probably the best-established environmental risk factor for dementia."

How to avoid injury and still stay active

- Know that walking out on an icy driveway in a cold winter can be dangerous. Many in the senior set wear Yak Tracks, tight little chains under your boots, a similar concept going back to the days when we attached chains to our car wheels. Another option is buying running shoes with built-in spikes driven into the soles.
- Take a defensive posture when there might be ice, a throw rug, or your grand kid's toys ahead. Anticipate, slow down, avoid or choose a safer route. Shamefully, I admit have much still to learn.
- Skis can be little vipers – they are slippery as hell. Other sports have risks but why avoid the sports you love? If you do not want to fall, do not ski, play tennis, pickle ball, or ride a road or mountain bike. Staying strong and agile is vital. Even walking down or up a curb can catch you unprepared, but falls are preventable. Exercise but be aware of the pitfalls.
-

How to:
- Do not think you can keep up with high schoolers.
- Watch out for your grandchildren's Legos, especially the ones with wheels. Get rid of throw rugs in the house.
- Work on balance. Work the Bosu ball. Watch Netflix while balancing on one foot to enhance your balance.

- Stay fit, strong, and agile. I am living proof that anyone can be a klutz and survive.

Anticipate. Think ahead: A boiler-plate solid, fail-safe way to avoid the preventable. Awareness on the front end can prevent negative outcomes on the back end.

Here are the components of balance:

Vision

Visual acuity is a vital part of the balance equation for men over 60. At a Saint Paul Chamber concert, I noticed the musicians were amber in my left eye, and clear in my right eye. The ophthalmologist confirmed I had two cataracts – the left worse than the right, and he would re-examine me in six months. I knew it would be only a matter of time before this ageing process worsened and my risk of falling could increase.

Vision determines how our body views the outside world. Peripheral vision, affected by retinal damage from diabetes or hypertension, if compromised, can be a dangerous invitation to miss unseen pets, slippery throw rugs, or unexpected curbs. Macular degeneration is the leading cause of loss of vision for individuals 50 years and older. Blood vessels that grow under the macula, can leak blood and fluid. Someone who is developing macular degeneration will first notice blurriness in the center of his vision. Next, there are wavy lines. Colors become washed out developing into blind spots. The process is called Wet Age-related Macular Degeneration.

Dr Leon, once a champion long distance runner and academic sports guru, once his macular degeneration progressed, adapted his exercise program to pole walking around the track at the University of Minnesota. Eventually, his ability to read and drive affected his mobility to commute, give slide presentations during lectures, and ultimately, enjoy his independence. Not for long. An innovative academician for over half a century, Professor Leon hired a driver to bring him back and forth from the university, and hiring a teaching assistant to present his slides.

Leon tells me how periodic intravitreal injections of "anti-VEGF", a curative drug inhibiting the formation of new blood vessels behind the retina, have maintained some of his vision. Without periodic injections, these vessels leak blood, lipids, and serum that permanently kill macular cells. Alternatively, ophthalmologists inject stem cells through the posterior chamber of the eye to replace supporting retinal pigment epithelium (RPE) with human embryonic stem cells. Leon takes his quadruple bypass and macular challenges in stride. "Art" literally walks the talk.

Since the cataract surgery in both of my eyes last summer, I cannot blame my vision any longer for going the wrong way in a cross-country ski race. Compromised vision has nothing to do with the litany of my falls. Failure not to anticipate my next step is the problem. I know I must focus before, during, and after I leap.

44

Proprioception

Proprioceptors are miniscule position receptors in our muscle spindles and joints that determine our spatial position in relation to gravity and the ground. Receptors, in our joints, feet, knees, hips, and torso, are another factor determining balance.

Proprioception assists us as we engage each step comprising gait. Proprioception controls the sensation of joint position in conjunction with vision and vestibular mechanisms as the significant ingredients for maintaining balance and ambulation. Men over 60 experience changes to proprioception as we do to similar age-related challenges of vision and the vestibular system increasing the risk of falling.

The Vestibular System: Everyone Needs a Gyroscope

The third determinant for successful balance is the vestibular complex comprised of the utricle, the saccule, and two semi-circular canals. The former two respond to acceleration. The vestibular system in the inner ear sends signals to the brain controlling balance and eye movements. The vestibular complex is complimentary to vision and proprioception for balance and mobility.

As I briefly explained regarding reasons for my falls, the three tiny semi-circular canals in each inner ear, are lined with sensory hairs that process motion, equilibrium, and spatial orientation. The vestibular complex controls eye movements and measures the gravitational, linear, and angular acceleration of the head in relation to inertial space.

The three interlocking rings are filled with tiny pebbles called ossicles and function like a gyroscope. The tiny stones called otoliths and fine hairs lining the canals sense position. If they are operating correctly, they keep us oriented in space. Debris that may collect inside the canals can lead to vertigo, dizziness, imbalance, spatial disorientation, visual disturbance, and even hearing loss. Someone with an inner ear dysfunction is unable to change positions without the world spinning out of control.

Vestibular dysfunction affects the eyes. We may be unable to properly focus. Someone with another inner ear challenge, tinnitus, is becoming ultra-sensitive to loud noises. Tinnitus, often associated with hearing loss, ringing, roaring, and buzzing in the ears can be a living hell. Sudden problems such as these are plenty reason to get medical advice.

Several years back, I experienced sudden dizziness while working out at the gym. Suddenly, my balance went haywire. I did not know why. I felt like I was on a Tilt-a-Whirl. A quick look up from touching my toes meant swaying with the world whirling around me.

I felt like vomiting. As a physician, I know too much. Said another way, I am as bad a hypochondriac as Woody Allen who, in Annie Hall, thinks a headache is a brain tumour. Give me a symptom and I fear the worst. In this case, I did not have an answer for my sudden dizziness, but I knew I needed to seek medical advice.

I was referred to a physical therapist who prescribed the Epley Manoeuvre, a series of fast position changes of the neck and head when rising quickly from lying supine to sitting up. In a percentage of cases this manoeuvre can correct benign paroxysmal positioning vertigo, which is what my doctor said I had. This technique of rapidly changing position works for some as it can retrain the semi-circular canals.

Unfortunately, my efforts to use the manoeuvre – moving my head from the horizontal to the upright position, made me nauseated and dizzier. So, why not do what works for ballet dancers? Now, after picking an object up from the floor, as I lift my head, I pick a spot twenty feet in front of me, focus on it, and it works. I am not dizzy.

After I presented the problem to the trainer at my gym, she recommended balancing on a Bosu Ball – a half-exercise ball on one side and a platform on the other. She had me balance first with two feet on the platform, then on one foot, touching the wall as needed. This manoeuvre has helped me the most to deal with my positional vertigo and movements I thought I would never be able to do again.

I still must focus on the clock on the wall in front of me. Now, I no longer need to hold her hand or the wall. Now, I can run from several feet away landing on the rubber ball side, begin jogging, and then balance on one foot even doing one or two-legged deep knee bends.

Using a Bosu ball is not for the faint of heart. Many have tried, many have failed. I am the envy of the over seventy set, sweating nearby on the elliptical But who, perhaps, wisely avoid working the Bosu as a way to improve their balance and agility. Their jealousy is palpable. But here is the good news. On steep downhills, I no longer become a trajectory into a snowbank.

I have made my ankles stronger by balancing on either side of the Bosu ball and I have avoided sprains and strains to my legs and ankles. Please, do not ask me to twirl on one foot at Yoga. I go down like a rock. Unfortunately, I lack the elasticity of my youth.

Gait, Posture and Locomotion

We have talked about balance. Now, let us talk about gait, posture, and locomotion. Soaring down cross-country tracks, I take precautions on sharp corners so I do not soar out of the track and into the woods. This is all about staying injury free. Cognition again.

Ageing presents its share of challenges. As described in the previous strength chapter, as we age over 60, we lose muscle mass. The name for this process again is sarcopenia. Losing proximal muscle strength can also makes it difficult getting up from a low chair or, God forbid, getting up from a fall.

Strengthening the small muscle in the ankles and feet with resistance exercises or on a Bosu ball helps us deal with unexpected changes in terrain. Examples include unexpectedly stepping on your grandson's ball on your walk to the bathroom or failing to see the curb. I have done them all and I am not even frail.

Joints may become arthritic as we age. Loss of earlier range of motion occurs with arthritic knees, wrists, or our neck as we age. No surprise, that sudden changes in position may contribute to a fall. A goal is to avoid going to ground. I made a bad decision not long ago as I was carrying a bag of salt down the front stairs planning to spread it around the garage apron. The stairs had a thin coat of ice. I slid down the stairs. That time I was lucky… no broken ribs.

Ageing men begin to feel it in their knees. Woe to the high school jock who got whacked high and low as he was tackled on the football field. Cleats can be a fulcrum. Goodbye meniscus. Although I played soccer into college, I never experienced such a cleat injury. My knees have not yet betrayed me despite years of running. Perhaps, in my favour is that I restrict my running to trails and as little as possible on pavement. I took time off from high intensity exercising from my 50s to my mid-60s. Consequently, I have had less wear and tear on my weight-bearing joints—knees, ankles, spine, and hips.

As I mentioned in the sex chapter, shoulder problems like a rotator cuff or previous dislocations can play havoc with your ability to hold yourself up in certain positions. I whine plenty about my rotator cuff or my AC separation. I have made a personal pledge that I will never go under the knife again in this lifetime, for a shoulder repair, specifically. Stretching and light hand weights used in Barre exercises have eliminated painful limitations moving my shoulders. Strengthening complimentary muscles around the shoulders, knees, neck, back, and core has important bearing on functions of gait, posture, and locomotion of these joints.

Strengthening opposing muscle groups enhances flexibility and improves how men over 60 accomplish activities of daily living (ADLs) including getting up off the Lazy Boy, toilet, or, God forbid, the floor. Complimentary exercises for all the major muscle groups benefit balance and gait. Consistent strength training makes such everyday tasks possible. We need pay special attention to strengthening proximal muscles like the quadriceps, the gluteals as well as strengthening our shoulders to complete essential tasks. Strong core strength enhances balance, posture, and gait. Crunches, if done carefully, will not injure your back. If it hurts, stop. Try a roller when you get up: a splendid way to massage your own back!

If you choose to be more aggressive, you can strengthen upper abdominal muscles as well you should, doing partial sit-ups on an incline board with or without the weight of your choice behind your neck. For the lower abdominals, try holding yourself up with your arms on a horizontal stationary bar, your feet dangling, while lifting your knees from vertical up to 45 degrees. Harder yet, is lifting your straight legs up to 45 degrees.

This is an easy prescription how you can strengthen the long muscles along your spine called the erector spinae that are essential for standing and walking. Here' a side tip: As an ageing senior, you should concentrate on maintaining an upright posture, understanding that good posture likes a strong back enhanced by good core strength. I have spoken about the possibility of and how to avoid senile posture. I advise not wearing ear buds on the bike path, or on the trail. We need all the cues of potential obstacles. Sudden changes in terrain or the unexpected biker or runner coming up fast on your right require vigilance and focus. Avoid distractions that might play havoc with balance, gait, and locomotion. Keep looking up!

When any of the three components of balance are compromised, taking a spill is a painful possibility. Anticipate the possibility of falling. Incidentally, knowing how to fall can save you from a more serious injury. As if you are a gaucho taking a tumble, and as if you flying off from a horse, there is the tuck and roll. Tuck in your arms, legs and head allowing the back of your shoulders and back to absorb the fall as you roll rather than stopping suddenly. Avoid an outstretched hand, arm, or your head. Better a thumb than a hip. But, worse yet, is a traumatic brain injury from a concussion, a brain bleed, or a subdural hematoma, as I experienced.

Exercise benefits flexibility, strength, posture, balance, and locomotion. The inevitable challenges of ageing can be delayed. The goal is growing older young. Or is it surviving growing older?

Chapter 5
Speed and Reaction Time

Exercise is an escape from stress. Men over 60 slow down. Slow-twitch outnumber fast-twitch muscle fibres enhancing endurance more than speed. Long slow workouts increase capillaries serving arms and legs improving oxygenation and performance. Exercise aerobically to a sweat thirty-minutes a day and add three strength workouts three or four days a week to build and maintain power. Carefully, chat with an exercise partner to avoid falling. Use a heart monitor if you wish. Take active rest days. This is about maintaining fitness but, most importantly, about having fun. Throw in bursts of high intensity intervals to enhance cardiac function. Forget "no pain no gain. Enjoy!". Unsure, find a personal trainer. If a woman(man)—and good—marry him/her.

"There is more to life than increasing its speed."

– Mahatma Gandhi

Here's a no brainer, who goes fastest, the old guys or the young guys? Why is that you may ask? Depends how long the race is. Young guys have more fast-twitch muscle fibres The over-60 set have more slow twitch fibres ergo, they are faster off the block for the 100; whereas, we can hold our own at the longer distances.

There is more awareness now how each age set excels in one speed or another: those of us over 60 - like you and me - excel in endurance. Athletes over 40 have taken their share of medals in marathons We need to adjust to our strong suit; that is, faster is not always better. This book's message is advocating consistency. Keep at it. We still can hold our own in the endurance race of life.

Nothing could have been better for the fitness movement than the innovation in the mid-70s of jogging. The movement put balance and fun to the aftermath of the Cold War. It became a wonderful opportunity for the young and old to attain cardiovascular fitness. The first man who made running popular, healthful, and desirable was running guru, Jim Fixx. America was receptive and bought more than a million copies of his book, *The Complete Book of Running* (1977). Overnight, his book leaped onto the New York Times Best Sellers. Fixx, in his books and on television talk shows, extolled the benefits of physical exercise and how it could extend life. The jogging movement was born.

The other savant who popularized the thrill of grabbing a pair of running shoes and taking to the pavement, was Dr George Sheehan, an eminent cardiologist from Rumson, N.J. Sheehan or "George," as he preferred to be called, was as much a philosopher as a champion master runner. His running manifesto, *Running and Being: The Total Experience* (1978) was also a runaway best seller.

He warned about retirement. "There are those of us who are always *about* to live. We are waiting until things change, until there is more time, until we are less tired, until we get a promotion, until we settle down-until, until, until. It always seems as if there is a major event that *must* occur in our lives before, we begin living."

He and Fixx popularised this simple form of exercise called "jogging", promising health, pleasure, and spirituality – the Zen of running. Their passion reached the young and old.

Not just a writing guru, Dr Sheehan, not only broke the five-minute mile record for men over 50 but took off on a personal mission for better health. His thoughts were apocryphal. America, young and old took to the streets. Despite that his prostate cancer had metastasised to his bones ten years later, he ran despite pain and discomfort. He only stopped when his strength gave out.

With a twinkle in his eyes, the thin and kindly running doctor advised, "Don't be concerned if running or exercise will add years to your life. Be concerned with adding life to your years." His parting words were apocryphal. "Humans come with a 75-year-old (body)." Ironically, he died a week short of this age. He kept running, speaking, and writing. I am 78 and the motor's still purring. I am not picking the year yet for my own departure. Why jinx a good thing.

Both running gurus reputedly attended the Mayo Clinic for medical evaluations. Shortly afterward, George began treatment for the prostate cancer discovered there. He listened, was treated, and his life was extended. Fixx may not have heeded medical advice to have further medical tests for suspected coronary artery disease. Unfortunately, earlier obesity and a three-pack -a-day smoking history and associated medical challenges, did not evolve as his apparent vigour had.

Fixx's demise was a sudden cardiac arrest while jogging on a rural Vermont road. The autopsy revealed three almost totally blocked coronary arteries. He had not listened to medical advice for intervention of a potentially life-threatening condition. The jogging both Fixx and Sheehan espoused had implicit virtue, but it is still vital to listen to your body as I fear Fixx did not.

If you have any risk factors such as a family history of heart disease, diabetes, hypertension, obesity, hypercholesterolemia, and are over 60, a physical could prolong your life. In my case, doctors had chosen not to treat my long-standing borderline elevated total cholesterol levels (over 200mg.%). In the midst of a tough life change, I developed transiently painful and apparent angina. Tests revealed I had correctable coronary occlusions. Mine were discovered in time. After finding the blockage, my cardiologist immediately implanted stents. Regrettably, Fixx did not choose this option. Two stents have provided 10 more active years for me, and I am still counting.

United we sit, so says avid athlete, Odd Osland. Society needs to get off its butt and, alone or in groups, get active. As we creep past 60, the goal must not be about achieving speed but, instead, developing and maintaining a pattern of consistency.

On my morning run – although for a shorter distance and at a lesser height than a soaring eagle, I feel like I am flying. After all, running is one of few sports when both feet are off the ground at one time. I have discovered the perfect antidote for whatever ails me, stress, ennui, boredom, or a house of noisy grandchildren. There may be other stressors to shake off: sending kids to college or earning for retirement. The story goes on and on and can refuse to quit if that is your choice. After I met this humble running hero after one of his lectures, Dr Sheehan, or "George" as he asked me at the time to call him, proved the quintessential runner, thinker, but primarily DOER. Imagine you are him as you set out for a run. I do.

Dr Sheehan did not spend unnecessary time waiting for retirement. He retired early to run, write, and motivate. His passion for running was for George Sheehan life itself. He lived life to the fullest but always in his own terms. Regardless of the season, the wind or cold blowing through his hair – he ran. His determination reminds me of the warning, "Men live lives of quiet desperation." No need to, brother.

George gave up a thriving medical career as a cardiologist to run, write, read, and speak relentlessly. His goal was to offer a multitude of running neophytes his vision how running could improve the quality of life as it had for him.

Age knows no limits. I have watched examples such as the Italian cross-country good medal relay champion Maurilio De Zolt, affectionately known as "The Cricket," five-foot plus some loose change, De Zolt took gold at 43.

He competed in cross-country skiing internationally from 1977 to 1997. At 43, De Zolt was the strong first leg on the 4X10 Italian relay team at the 1994 Winter Olympics in Lillehammer that trounced the Norwegians on their own turf by less than a tenth of a second. Norway went into mourning after being beaten in their national sport by Italians. All Norway was on suicide watch I suspect.

I want Maurilio's élan. We are both short… and fast. I too want to be the fastest skier in my age group. Reality bite One: With age there is a dwindling number of competitors in my age group. Reality bite two: it is not how good an athlete you are, but who shows up on race day.

Over 60 now, Maurilio looks younger than most men half his age. When asked in an interview after he had retired from competition as to what he attributes his long success as a racer? He laughs. "Red wine and pasta." Spoken like a true Italian.

Most men over 60 DO have the juice to begin exercising after an appropriate medical check-up. My running coach answered my question of how to excel. "Take a chance. Smell the flowers. Crest don't rest. Start strong and finish stronger. Start slow but be persistent." Let your motor run a bit as you check your balance, flexibility, and strength. They should all fit nicely together. There are no limits that are not possible by adhering to a realistic exercise program that may defy societal misconceptions of our ability. Sceptical? Do not hesitate to consult a certified exercise specialist or a physically active physician.

Once we pass 50, response and reaction time do slow. I am aware when I ski race, for instance, I need to set my expectations around my own age group. However, I still recall the shock, even sadness, when a friend over 60, realised he could no longer break into the first 100 in a prestigious race as he had consistently managed over the past decades.

SJ Perelman described so aptly how age affects us in *Under the Spreading Atrophy* before academics coined the word, "sarcopenia". With proper nutrition, strength, and speed training, we have a better chance of closing the ageing gap or, at least, keep up with our same-aged friends.

There is one shocking story after another of someone in their late seventies, who, we suspect, thought he could cross a set of railroad tracks quickly enough to avoid an oncoming train. I keep asking myself, did he think he could outrun the train? Reaction time slows. We may have less attuned visual or auditory cues Studies show that individuals over 60 compensate in favour of safety. They are certainly more careful than testosterone-laden younger drivers. Over 60, we must avoid cognitive errors that result in accidents and can be avoided. Think first, step second.

Cognitive behavioural skills – let us call them a greater awareness of our speed and reaction time that can prevent avoidable consequences. How fast we can react over 60 may make the difference between crossing the train tracks intact or becoming an engine ornament.

Tad Friend, in a recent New Yorker article, tells how the elders at the other side of the squash court time-lapsed before him… "Graying and thickening, face shields, elbow sleeves, and knee braces." He notices, among the 14 guys in their 70s, only two can still sprint. My observations of the 85-plus group in most races is, no entrants. The winner by default is age.

As balance and mobility diminish, self-confidence can as well. As a result, many no longer wish to participate. But there is always some 90-year-old Chinese lady from Queens who still manages to run a credible Boston Marathon. Oh, she always takes her age group… and, in that iconic race, especially, she's still got some tough competition.

At our age, what is the difference between a nice trip to the supermarket or a driving accident? Neurobiological changes can cause response delay, compromised speed, and delayed reaction time. Does thirsting to ski race suggest I have a death wish? I may just be choosing one of the two ways I want to die. The other one begins in a horizontal position. The disastrous fall and near-death subdural practicing for an upcoming ski race a few years back almost confirmed the other choice, in a ski race. The former, perhaps of lesser danger (in the past, mind you), would be in the sack but, hopefully, not after being caught by the lovely lady's irate husband. Crucial: I do not want a slow, painful, or lingering death. Either option ensures none of the above.

My colleague, Ernie, a general surgeon of excellent repute, told me he had recently retired. I was shocked. As we chatted, he looked at his hands as he answered my question, "Why did you stop as a surgeon?" He quietly answered my question, "I didn't think I could take the risk any longer. I decided to retire at the top of my skill set."

"How young are you?" I asked. His answer surprised me because he looked 60. "I'm 77." But then, my friend then told me how he has rediscovered himself by adapting to what he perceived could be potential limitations. He described how he had turned a liability into an asset. "I supervise, on a part-time basis, a Suboxone(buprenorphine) and methadone program at a drug treatment clinic." He may no longer trust his hands, but his success at a new parttime medical challenge has made him stay vital. Others regrettably needed a not-so-subtle nudge to lay down the stethoscope.

As we age, our response time slows. Accepting this can be difficult. Taking longer to get a job done as quickly as our younger co-workers can be humiliating and threaten job security especially when it affects our employer's bottom line. A higher pay scale for an older employee due to longevity compared with a more affordable up-and-coming new colleague who can start at a lower pay scale, may spell the adage, "In with the new, out with the old." Judged by our age or influenced by society's perceptions of our limitations can spell move-over-time for gray beard. More about retirement in the next chapter.

Understanding the complexities of the new computerised technology can be a deal breaker for someone over 60. Many older physicians faced with the new electronic medical record (EMR) retired early. As an intern at Johns Hopkins Bayview, I remember documenting on call many endless nights histories and physicals on too many patients on my small portable typewriter. How technology has changed.

Fast forward in careers after I had left medicine in my early 60s, I applied and was hired to do chemical health assessments as a licensed alcohol and drug counsellor at a treatment program. I struggled getting up to speed with the new templates I used for the evaluations. In my own mind, I developed speed and efficiency. But, alas, not fast enough for my first supervisor. At the end of my first week, the person from human services who had hired me, called apologetically, and broke the bad news for this oldster. "The clinic is letting you go. It just doesn't seem to be working out." A more accurate but illegal announcement might have been, "You're fired, old guy!"

Men over 60 show variability in mastering new intellectual challenges. One 65-year-old competitor – active and fit – continues to blow away younger competitors. His successes contradict most statistics. The reality of ageing can be hurtful and, as in his case that I described earlier, humiliating. Later, my friend, despite Herculean accomplishments, has had to accept the challenge of ageing based on the speed at which he can "turn it over" an unlikely to still be top dog.

Ageing affects individuals differently. Dr Michael DeBakey had a career spanning 75 years. He pioneered innovative and life-saving surgical procedures well into his 80s. Jascha Heifetz, considered by many the greatest violinist of all time, adapted to his ageing evolution by turning to teaching and social causes. Wilhelm Kempff, the renowned pianist of his day, excelled through his 60s and well into his 80s. The longevity Kempff demonstrated was an amalgamation of fine motor skills, coordination, and speed. By his own admission, he practiced endlessly. These maestros advocate, "Practice, Practice, Practice."

Such examples of enduring cognitive-behavioural abilities are an endorsement for sweat and repetition. I hate the word luck. Certainly, great genes and an artistic or athletic gift, can complement exhaustive practice. The DeBakey's, the Heifetz's, the Kempff's bring many components to their remarkable longevity. Persistence and discipline account to much of their success. Let us call it refusing to give up.

About to undergo the repair of two cataracts, for a fleeting moment, I wondered if I should entrust my cataract surgery to the youthful 77-year-old ophthalmologist I had chosen. Not acquiring points for tact, I asked him how he felt about his abilities at 77. His assurance became my reassurance. "I feel 100%," he told me with a smile. He repaired both cataracts flawlessly.

There is variability of response rates for those over 60 derived from evidence-based data. What is my eye doctor's success rate? How does he fare in the OR, or more importantly, how do his patients fare? What do the OR nurses have to say about him? I knew his record is flawless. Lest I fell prey to the same ageism I have experienced, I trusted Bob's repetitive and enduring successful cataract surgeries. His evident skill set confirms his abilities. Bob tells me though, he knows when he will stop.

My professional musician friends tell me that they attribute their successful performances and artistic skills to hard, long practice, and performing. They tell me that, although they may be in the twilight of their careers, they practice more, not less. Experts attribute continuing stellar artistic performances to brain plasticity in an older performer that is very much enhanced by long practice sessions.

There are other ways ageing artists keep achieving. Some find joy complementing professional artistry with joyous passions. For instance, my dear friend, Julia Bogorad-Kogan, the long-time St Paul Orchestra ("SPCO") flutist, has danced ballet for decades. Chuck, Ullery, now retired from his chair as the SPCO principal bassoonist, to his delight, has taken up weight training and aerobic activities that he is certain have enhanced his strength, vitality, and contentment.

What we who are over 60 should be concerned about is how fast we can react to an errant driver fantasising he is Mario Andretti especially, when he chooses to run a red light while we are in the middle of the intersection. Aware of the inevitable changes of how I will react to a distracted driver, I let others weave around me. I drive slower and more defensively. I try not to react when another speedster like our NASCAR wannabe, hangs on my back fender. I avoid using my cell phone except for navigation but, even that, carefully.

Dr Art Leon explains that the brain has plasticity that compensates for the sensorimotor decline of ageing. When is it time to get the car keys away from an increasingly frail 80-year old mother or grandparent? Such an allusion of agelessness may be a liability. An intervention if we are concerned about dad's cognitive or physical competency, is a painful act of love by a concerned family member. Unexplained accidents, getting lost while out driving with brittle diabetes, or failing the vision screening at the DMV, are realistic reasons for grandpa to surrender his driver license. At a certain age, the department of motor vehicles may require an updated driving competency and vision test.

"Driving represents freedom, mobility, and autonomy." Spirduso notes: "Driving an automobile is a psychomotor skill... that most adolescents passionately desire to learn and that almost all ageing adults dread."

Driving a vehicle is a psychomotor skill that requires perceptual ability, vigilance, short-and long-term memory, and motor programming. If all else fails, give me a call when your 90-year-old grandmother has taken the car out to visit the casino or a trip to the grocery store. Perhaps, this is a time to stay off the road until granny gets home.

Chapter 6
Retirement – Good News or Bad News

Retirement, the hardest hurdle, is the opportunity for a man over 60 to redefine himself and renew self-worth. "Who am I?" We now search for our essence. We struggled to provide. Now, we must find own gold.

The cultural impact of retirement is second only to health concerns in men over 60. We face mortality. Many may die soon after retirement succumbing to illness or declining health. "I am no longer important. No one knows me in retirement," An man or woman might exclaim. Perhaps to hide his fear, a friend laughs, "I don't mind retirement. It's what comes next that concerns me." Prepare for retirement and maximise the opportunity to rediscover yourself.

"We retire too early, and we die too young. Our prime of life should be in the 70's and old age should not come until we are almost 100."

– Joseph Pilates, "Contrology"

Retirement can be an exciting time. Perhaps, for the first time, we can now have the leisure and freedom to travel freely or pursue other interests and bucket lists. We can finally slow down and smell the flowers. But, for many men both the anticipation and reality of retirement can be challenging, even intimidating. The adjustment to the loss of a work routine and a sense of purpose can leave a vacuum in our souls.

Retirement can bring new relationship challenges. Men who do not find meaningful replacement for their work identities may have a sense of purposelessness. What may begin as boredom can lead to depression and even health problems. Men in retirement must redefine their sense of self. Suddenly, even overnight, how we define ourselves must shift from WHAT I do to WHO I am.

This is the time when a man must interpret self-worth less by what he has done in the workplace for the past 40 years but, now must search deep inside for his elusive essence and what The Mankind Project, The New Warriors Training Adventure, calls finding a man's gold. such a transition splashes cold onto our face with the question, "Who am I?" The achievement of self-acceptance is one of the great gifts of later life. Hopefully, we can say, "I am now an elder and I am proud of it."

Erik Erikson explains that the seventh stage of our lives is one of ego integrity. This stage of our life is no longer about empire building. Kids have long since left the house. We have phased out of our working life. Now, we can evaluate our accomplishments over our life. Now, there are grandchildren enrolled in college or are playing endless games of soccer or baseball for us to watch. Many of our dearest friends may still be available for an afternoon coffee. All too many are gone. That we appreciate a sense of closure and completeness is preferable to feeling depressed that we have failed to have made a significant contribution to society.

As we stand around at reunions, old friends describe 40 years of a happy marriage. I am a bit suspicious on that one. Others share the happiness of a successful second marriage. It is inevitable that we will share our feelings about those who have already passed. What we may not want to talk about is the tension that may have come to our primary relationship. We may struggle how now we may be perceived by our partner as "getting under foot," especially if our wives are also at home. We may bring a lowered self-esteem to the breakfast table. We are no longer a top gun lawyer, a phenomenal brick layer, or the go-to accountant. We are no longer the primary bread winner, but now maybe on a $1500 a monthly social security check.

Loneliness and isolation often accompany ageing. he friends still in our lives are dying, have moved south, or just losing mobility. I have found several friends who, despite our wonderful high school, college, or medical school relationships, no longer correspond. Is it that a retired friend has lost self-esteem, preferring to project silence as his way of hiding insecurity or embarrassment

None of us are who we were decades ago. Much time at my fiftieth college reunion was about reminiscence. The majority wore masks of contentment rather than what was under it – a fear-as my buddy joked-about what comes next.

A man over 40, who is widowed or divorced later in life, now must whip up dinner for one, run a few pairs of underwear through the washing machine and dryer, or keep up with bills his partner handled before; His departed wife may have done the "heavy lifting" around the house. Responsibilities that were deferred to our mates, are now ours to do.

Jessica Bruder in *The End of Retirement* (Harper's Magazine, August 2014), relates,

"After the age of 60 has been reached, the transition from non-dependence to dependence is an easy stage – property gone, friends passed away or removed, relatives (have) become few, ambition collapsed, only a few short years left to live, with death a final and welcome end to it all – such conclusions inevitably sweep the wage earner from hopeful independent citizen into that of the helpless poor."

She tells how many seniors who, for financial reasons, must postpone retirement and drive into the sunset as the new migrant workers, "Nomads" on the mobile home circuit. Despite physical limitations from chronic problems such as arthritic hips or knees, they have become the new migrant worker. Now, parttime workers for big box stores, they may walk endless distances from one end of these huge stores to the other, endure repetitive assembly lines, or shelve heavy loads of freight. These may be jobs for which they are physically unqualified. Yet, they need the money.

They could call themselves the gray "Oakies" of the new recession. Many are seniors who lost their savings in the 80s and 90s. It is easy for them to question, "Are these our Golden Years?" One could argue that their engagement in the work force may help them feel vital and needed. Of course, there are always grandchildren to care for knowing that we can go home after our shift.

Mark Luborsky in the December 2003 issue of *Cross-Cultural Gerontology* asks if people in all cultures retire? Historically and cross-culturally, the practice of retirement may be anything but common. "The 21st century is no longer about farmers and craftsmen proud of the work that defined them. With the advent of industrialisation, it is now all about an age-fixed, socially mandated final phase in a career of employment."

With the advent of the electronic medical record (EMR) an age-related transformation has had a major impact on my profession, medicine, as well as with a myriad of other advocations. Replacing the over-60 worker with younger workers may be related to the perceived notion we have significant declining speed or reaction time. Perhaps, we have become too expensive.

Many senior physicians moved aside when they could not tackle the electronic medical record (EMR). They went peacefully but, in a certain way, tragically. Such precipitous retirement can contribute to our loss of purpose when we lose the opportunity to share our wisdom as an elder.

William Graebner and Jill Guadagno explain, "Retirement is a rarity in tribal and village society." The Eskimos, historically, sent the frail elderly off on the closest departing ice flow. Hypothermia, luckily, is reputedly a painless death. That is, if you believe there is a nice way to die. Let me know if you do.

Is there a pattern we men over 60 share as age closes in? We are now gray. Our skin can be wrinkled. We are slower off the starting block. Maybe, we can be a tad more confused and, worse yet, more forgetful. "Why did I come upstairs?" faced with less work cues, it is not unusual to ask, "Is it Monday or Tuesday?"

It does not necessarily follow that we all will have a financial safety net after retirement. Some politicians talk of ending social security – already a pittance— and, for many, and often well below the poverty level. The same lawmakers appear to shrug off the current health challenge of an escalating aging population rather than making it better for the older citizen. They would slash funds for the disadvantaged or those with pre-existing illnesses.

How does Ayn Rand's so-called rugged individualism apply to growing old? I am not so sure how an increasingly industrialised and electronically driven society has carved a rewarding place for elders as they appear to enjoy in less developed countries. In Andean culture, the concept of retirement is unknown. Among the Aymara of Bolivia, Southern Peru, and Northern Chile, the elderly stay active until death.

In 1946, L.W Simmons in the *Journal of Gerontology*, described how life in primitive societies was short. Relatively few ever reached old age let alone what, in modern societies, was later coined "retirement". Able to survive the rigors of primitive life, those ageing in such cultures reputedly remained more vigorous than those of us in modern society. The elderly remained a valuable part of society. "They are regarded as repositories of knowledge, imparters of valuable information, and mediators between their fellows and the fearful supernatural powers." Simmons adds, "The proportion… who remain active, productive, and essential… is much higher than in advanced civilisations… giving the old person a greater chance to be regarded as a treasured asset."

Flash forward to the here and now. My dear professional musician friend, Chuck, the principal bassoonist of 40 years for the world-renowned SPCO, recently retired, quipped, "A big component of my self-worth has been being part of the orchestra." His are a litany of the pros and cons of retirement.

"How does your age figure in?" I ask.

He turns toward me and, with a cupped hand to his left ear, confides his hearing is bad in that ear.

"I've had some health issues. I am trying out a new hearing aid. I have had some heart problems including atrial fibrillation which has significantly affected how much I can do. I had an ablation for it recently. I had a transient ischemic attack (TIA) not long ago and, for a couple of hours, lost my vision. I'm on a blood thinner for both problems."

I admire how Chuck can share such jolting physical challenges and that he has bravely pushed forward.

"I know more about how to play. I know how the music should sound. To accomplish how I had performed over the past forty years, I found it harder and more stressful. I found I had to practice much more. Maybe, I am more thoughtful about my playing. I think about the music more. I generally found I was able to compensate. I found I could not always count on my reflexes as I did when I was 25. I found I had to prepare more. I needed to figure out where things could go wrong. I stopped teaching hoping there would be less danger of shorting myself or burning out."

"You've taught for some time, haven't you?" I ask.

He lists places he has mentored aspiring musicians.

"I was teaching at the University of Minnesota but stopped doing that some time ago. I tell students that very few can reach professional musician status and I spent a lot of time coaching them about other career possibilities. I try to help them think about alternatives to performing professionally in an orchestra as I have done and where jobs are scarce. Originally, I was a mathematician but, gravitated to the SPCO from the army band."

"I asked myself, "Do I want to stay and die on the job, or should I retire?"

Finally, I decided that by retiring, I could catch up on my reading, visit the kids and grandkid, and clean the house." I understood how Chuck was alluding to the challenges men have as they approach and, finally, enter retirement. The questions Chuck expresses are about knowing that such a sequence he describes is not imaginary, and that the next phase of our lives may not be Valhalla, but rather carry the risk of emptiness. We need to locate the parachute to contentment.

Men, now in the aftermath of a brilliant career like Chuck, must now deal with vulnerability. He and his wife, an equally accomplished violinist who had been with the chamber for 40 years as well, together, stood at the edge of the stage after their final performance to accept the accolades of the orchestra president and the standing ovation of an adoring audience bidding them farewell.

Their mutual retirement testifies how they will support one another. I sense Chuck's resolution to take on the challenges of retirement will enhance his transition from performer to living a different yet equally fulfilling life. He tells me they have many common interests and are best friends. Unfortunately, so many of us may experience loneliness despite a lifelong marriage and partnership. The danger is that when the time arrives, we may isolate. Men are reticent to ask for help. We may be ashamed to expose our soft underbelly.

"This is good. This is good,' Chuck reassures me. 'I have been with the orchestra 40 years. Both my wife and I have really done a lot for it. I have shaped the organisation. I feel happy now about our mutual decision to retire.'"

Yet, I sense a tone of sadness that he has decided to sever ties from what has been for almost a half century, his extended family.

Our conversation then moved into even more serious territory.

"Ageing that is happening to me, portends the frailty that ultimately comes to all of us," he tells me. "I am considering my options. Just as my father did, I have gotten everything together, so I won't be a burden for my own children."

Chuck seems wistful as he describes his own father's death three years before.

"My brother and I took turns traveling to Tucson to look in on him. What was so beautiful was that he wanted to make his passing easy for us. He prepared everything: his service, his obituary. He prepaid his funeral expenses. I will admit what he did made me sad. Some of what he did seemed morbid to me. At his request, we had morphine just in case his prostate cancer became too painful. We did not have to resort to that. He died as I was getting on the plane to see him again. It was as if he had planned it that way."

The challenge posed by retirement occurs the minute we punch out for the last time from a career that has defined us. We are exuberant. "Free at last". This may be the first time that many of us must explore what our essence is – who we really are. Now, we risk falling into an abyss that could await us as we enter the next phase of our lives. We risk losing a sense of identity attached to what we did.

Someone I met soon after I had retired asked, "What do you do?"

Predictably, I answered, "I used to be a doctor."

Now, wait a minute – once a doctor, always a doctor. Now, without the trappings of respect given a professional, I needed to dig deep for the power to replace outward definitions of myself with my realness, my goodness, or, as the New Warriors of the Mankind project describe, as my gold".

Now, I am just another anonymous author grinding out a book at Dunn Brothers that is now, my "office". The rent is cheap but secretarial help can be hard to find. My productivity is now defined by my writing, ski racing, coaching, and my new pleasure, as a house husband who does all the shopping, cooking, cleaning, and other work around the house.

Men may have an unconscious fear about leaving the working world. There is no longer a work routine. We risk losing a sense of purpose. Discovering how to fill leisure time can become work. "Do I have to play golf again?" could be the refrain those on the front end of retirement never expected to ask. Retirement can be an exciting time. A man over 60, finally has the leisure time for travel or to fulfil passions long deferred by responsibility.

Retirement may bring new relationship issues. A spouse now discovers she has a needy husband underfoot, who may be unable to find meaningful activities. The new danger can be boredom, a sense of purposelessness, depression, or unexpected health problems.

Retirement time can be a dangerous point in a man's life. The two most risky times for suicide among us over 60 can be early retirement or after losing a spouse of many years. The rate of suicide doubles between 65 and 85. As explained in *Dr D's Handbook for Men Over 40, a Guide to Fitness, Health, Living and Loving in the Prime of Life*, women try, men do. Statistically, men over 74 have the highest risk for suicide. Typically, women will admit they are depressed while most men "tough it out". An older woman will see their doctor. We have a few drinks and then pull the trigger.

One Man's Bucket List

Now for a couple personal retirement stories. One of my lifelong fantasies was to hang out for a summer restoring a boat, watching incomparable sun rises and sets, billowing clouds off the stern, and shifting weather. So, here's the story. Retired, my life is now unencumbered. It does not get any better than that. It is eight in the morning, and the inhabitants on other boats are just waking up. I am leaning up against the wheelhouse, the front deck is cluttered with sanders, paint cans, and extension cords. I am wearing paint-covered Bermudas, and a floppy "T" shirt – tanned from head to toe, steaming coffee in hand – watching the sun coming up over the distant Apostle islands and Lake Superior.

Feeling the moment, as the sun is rising, I am a symbol of freedom to those poor souls lined up on the pier waiting to take the tour boat around the Apostles. They are still worker bees and unable yet to partake of one perk of retirement; that is, free time accompanied with great health. I know I am an object of admiration, regardless of my age, among those counting the days until retirement.

The owner of the boat had offered an exchange of free rent and a summer living on the boat in return for sweat equity; sanding, caulking, and painting. He even threw in the scraper, power sander, and paint. I am aboard the slave ship. For the next 3 months it was just me and my senses spirited by a daily cold shower from the hose next to the boat, all the fresh fish I could eat from the boats a block away by the docks, and maybe, best of all, getting rocked to sleep every night inside the breakwater. Strong black coffee in hand on the poop(ed) deck, it is now late afternoon, and the sun is setting. I take in a 150-degree panorama of Basswood, Stockton, Hermit, and Madeline islands, four of many that comprise The Apostle Island National Lakeshore.

To a few who walked by and were curious about what I was doing, I would say, "Want a tour of the boat?"

My guests, after they heard that I was no longer working and was retired, would say, "Wow, you really are lucky." I didn't tell them the old tank leaked like a sieve.

That gave my ego a zip. In their mind, they were visiting an adventurous septuagenarian dispelling a common notion that retirement must be clouded in loneliness and uselessness rather than a time of vigour.

'How old do you think I am?' I often asked.

Fortunately, most guessed low, but I suspect some did so to compliment my lifestyle and not my age. We can fulfil our dreams. Perhaps, a few realised from my happiness that retirement can be less about lost identity and more about what is the next challenging event.

I hoped that among those who passed by as I was sanding a rail or patching a hole in the bridge that they might become more optimistic about what lies ahead at the end of their anticipated seven years, one month, two weeks, twenty minutes, and thirty-five seconds before they retire. Focus on your gold, your essence, your passion. Explore who you really are so you can make the best use of the next exciting and fulfilling stage in front of you.

A Finn Whose Entire Life Takes on Bucket Lists

Juho, a Minnesota River Valley transplant, originally from Finland, and well into his 60s, came to the rich black Minnesota River farmland in his 40s and is now well over retirement age. The tall, gangly farmer just won't quit. As we sit chatting in his loft office above his pole barn, soft rain is pinging off the metal roof. I quickly realise his life has always been a whirl of challenge not unlike the delicate flutter of a butterfly as it passes from flower to flower. As he quietly explains the adventures and accomplishments of his life, I am amazed that anyone could do so much in one lifetime. Juho's life belies the word, "retirement".

The stories of his many lifetime journeys that he shared with me are awesome. In his lilting Finnish accent, he tells me, "Once the farming was over for the season, I bicycled 3000-miles from the farm, across the country, over the Tetons, and through Mexico. I always felt safe." He delights telling me more about other thousand-mile bike trips to the Yucatan on his favourite well-worn bike against the wall beside him. Juho is a man of physical accomplishments. He shares, "I have done a few marathons, but I could never train hard enough because of the demands of spring planting and the fall harvest. I just do not have the time these days to take those long trips. I visit Finland quite a bit when I'm not delivering grain around here during the winter."

Thin, tall, and animated, Juho tells me about one book or another he is currently reading, and his passionate commitment helping needy countries. That he now into his late 60s does not appear to have slowed him down. Humbly, he tells me about his passion providing trucks he finds that he then repairs and brings to third-world countries like Haiti. "The real impact that motivates me will be bringing reverse osmosis to such needy countries." He repairs every type of farm implement his neighbours are unable to fix.

He tells me of his concern that the constant rain this spring will affect his planting. "You know, the one thing we have no control over is Mother Nature. We can try to control people around us but never nature." What he tells me reminds me how little control we have as we pass 60. Juho shows no signs of slowing down. He may be the only farmer in the Valley who, after the planting is done for the day, bikes home from a distant rented field.

He and his second wife, a commuting non-profit administrator, delight in each other's company enjoying a log home he brought log-by-log from Finland. Their rural paradise is situated by driving down a steep hill through an original hardwood forest. He tells me about his unique "smoke" sauna off the lower pasture, and a wood sauna next to his lap pool in the lower level of his house.

Juho abounds with energy. His life defines a vitality that can morph into active retirement. Yet, he laments his own ageing process. "I don't have the strength I once had. There was the time when I easily handpicked fields of sweet corn." Replacing earlier cross-country bike trips, he now devotes energy toward building a new home – one boulder and one log at a time, above the Black River in Colorado. His dedication to wanderlust and adventure refuses to quit because they define his life. This is the same farmer who once ski trekked across Finland to Sweden. He does not show any evidence of quitting and seems always searching for the next peak to summit. Retirement for Juho will clearly not be as most men over 60 define it.

Another Man Who Defies Stereotypes of Ageing

Milton Harrison, a long-time gym friend, is a 70-year-old African American who refuses to follow expected stereotypes of ageing or being Black. A few years back, I met Milton for the first time in the locker room at the community centre. We chatted as we changed and when I asked what he had studied in college, he told me he had a master's degree in French literature.

What Milt told me after we became gym friends confirmed he is no stranger to athletic prowess. A quintessential collegiate track athlete, he won the first Brooklyn Marathon. "I play to win," He assured me.

Early success through the New York Road Runners Club led to a cross-country scholarship to Wayne State. His athletic accomplishments are legendary. He was a Golden Gloves boxer, started on the wrestling team, and excelled in the relay, the high jump, triple jump, and the one mile run at Wayne State. He was second man on the WSU cross-country team and had a 3.5 grade point average. He also told me how he dealt with blatant prejudice toward Black students. "Those were unfriendly times for young Black students at Midwestern colleges," Milt explained. Despite adversity, "Milt" has always given of himself.

After graduations, he taught at a Minneapolis inner-city high school, all the while boxing competitively. Milton later joined the YMCA and quickly climbed their career ladder, all the time finding the time to train and race including winning the first Twin Cities Marathon. Milton later travelled east to become the director at the Newark YMCA which was at the time struggling.

With a great deal of pride, Milton tells me, 'Hell, they've even got a street named after me in Newark.' Harrison set up the first Sports Legends Program giving inner city kids access to famous athletes who showed them that a great athlete believed in them and that they had the ability to also succeed.

When Milton retired from his career back east at the "Y," it just was a few months before he became bored and took a job as an administrator for a senior care community. In 2012, he gathered a veritable who's who of sports greats for The Sports Legends Extravaganza Charity Golf Tournament to raise money so that "… those in society who are in need are not forgotten."

When I see him at the gym, Milton is always smiling and mellow. He reliably sweats up a storm but still schmoozes with all his gym buddies. He and his four senior co-exercisers are lined up on exercycles laughing and reliably giving me grief whenever I pass by on my way to barre with the gals, or moving toward. the free weights. After we both finish our workouts and are changing from our gym clothes, Milton, gets ready to go as he straightens his tie and pulls on a well-fitting sport coat. He tells me he is heading for a breakfast meeting and quips, "Continuing staying fit is vital." For Milton, the pace has slowed, but, in his late 70s, he maintains a consistent dedication to fitness.

When I look up from tying my shoes, I realise that Milton has quietly slipped away for his first meeting of the day.

Chapter 7
Spirituality – Where Is God When We Need Him

Rites, rituals, and ceremonies define our values. They define us. They reflect what we value, and who we are. Reverend Gere defines the spiritual within the physical, and not a stage of survival. The spiritual is our world view. Physical health and spiritual health can live in harmony by balancing body and spirit, and finding harmony, tranquillity, peacefulness, and serenity as well as grace, perspective, patience, and acceptance. We now represent wisdom. Be still and look inward for self-identity. Rediscover core traditions and holiness in others and ourselves. Weep first. Then laugh as laughter can heal anguish and despair. Living finds its completion in dying.

"Nobody grows old merely by living a number of years. We grow old by deserting our ideals. Years may wrinkle the skin, but to give up enthusiasm wrinkles the soul."
– Samuel Ullman, Poet "Youth", 1914

I am pleased to write this chapter of *Handbook for Men over 60: Don't Quit Now!* linking the spiritual dimension of living and ageing to the physical. The author and I knew each other as young men in college hurdling the 20-year-old mark. That was 50 years ago. Each in our own way-he in the field of medicine, I as a clergyman-have learned that bodies and souls, inextricably linked, take a beating–often severe–throughout life's journey.

We would agree that we have at least as many scars as medals to show for our life's efforts. We have discovered that the broken heart and the seared soul have been more effective mentors in preparing us for the future than a victory lap before an adoring crowd. Yet, even with past as prologue, we strive for more years of life and the experiences – both sweet and bittersweet.

We are convinced that those who take care of both the physical and the spiritual dimensions of their lives after 60 can do more than survive. During this season of life, people can thrive! As a Presbyterian pastor, I have been privileged to be with people at their times of greatest joy and deepest sorrow. I have joined with them at mountain top moments of life and slogged with them through their valleys, shrouded in death's shadow. I have been present at births and deaths, and every conceivable occasion in between. Each event has pointed me to a timeless reality spoken by the preacher of long ago whose words are recorded in the Book of Ecclesiastes. *"For everything there is a season, and a time for every matter under heaven."*

The preacher illustrates this profound truth revealed during the seasons and times of life this way:

A time to be born, and a time to die.
A time to plant, and a time to pluck up what is planted.
A time to kill, and a time to heal.
A time to break down, and a time to build up.
A time to weep, and a time to laugh.
A time to mourn, and a time to dance.
A time to throw away stones, a time to gather stones together.
A time to embrace, and a time to refrain from embracing.
A time to seek, and a time to lose.
A time to keep, and a time to throw away,
A time to tear, and a time to sew.
A time to keep silence, and a time to speak.
A time to love, and a time to hate.
A time for war and a time for peace.

The preacher then leaves his hearers with this question. *What gain have the workers from their toil?* Our answer depends upon how our spiritual life informs our general outlook on life. Matters of the spirit determine how we view the world and those with whom we share our life's journey. Such realities as seeking and losing, keeping, and throwing away, apply to all aspects of life; physical, intellectual, psychological, and spiritual.

The mind or psyche and the body, or soma, are partners in our lives. Physical health and spiritual health are most fully
achieved when they live in harmony within us. Of course, one mode prevails, depending upon age and situation. "Mind over matter" can be helpful in shaking off fatigue to finish a project, or to keep us from succumbing to unhealthy, worldly self-indulgences. Conversely, to the person who says, "I'd rather wear out than rust out," the cautionary tale is that what sets us humans apart from the rest of the creatures in the Creation is not our physical attributes so much as our ability to think and reason, and feel deep-seated emotions.

Physicality dominates the seasons of our earlier years. Much of a child's work is kinaesthetic play. Adolescence, while emotion-laden, presents itself with great physical change at the onset of puberty. Throughout one's 20s and 30s, barring an unforeseen condition or traumatic injury, the human body functions with "all systems go" as its watchword.

Then comes the realisation that the author pointed out in his *Handbook for Men Over 40*. The length and quality of the remaining seasons of our lives depends in great measure on our taking time to balance the needs and realities of our bodies and our spirits.

One's personal prologue for any *Handbook for Men Over 60* is assessing how life has been lived in the time zone of one's 40s and 50s. The prologue for this is a man's 20s and 30s. For me, even though I was active in the "religion business" throughout my 20s and 30s, I could not find a balance between the physical and the spiritual in the seasons of my life until I came to grips with my declining physical prowess.

My first true awareness of internalising this new season in my life happened just before I turned 40. Always athletic, I was a sports-obsessed child. I learned to read by poring over the sports section of the daily paper. Given a choice of topics for an English theme, I wrote about sports. Growing up on a bucolic college campus in the innocent days of the 1950s, my friends and I had unlimited access to mowed and lined sports fields complete with soccer and lacrosse goals in season, a hockey rink, a gymnasium, tennis courts, and a golf course. Every day after school, and every possible hour on weekends, my friends and I were shooting hoops or pucks in one of these palaces, or running in pursuit of a ball on these sacred grounds. To me, the setting was paradise.

My self-identification as an athlete, fuelled by the perception of those who knew me, continued throughout college and graduate school, as I played sports as an undergraduate and then coached intercollegiate hockey. Inevitably, that season in my life ended, and, ready or not – I needed to embrace a new season. The matter under heaven I had to deal with was recognising that I had literally "lost a step physically".

Unless one suffers a sudden, traumatic injury before "losing a step" – think a torn ACL or a ruptured Achilles tendon – the loss is gradual, almost imperceptible, throughout one's 20s and 30s. Then, one day it happens. The forms and settings are many and varied, but the reality is the same for all.

For me, the recognition that I had "lost a step" occurred during our annual neighbourhood Fourth of July parents vs. kid's soccer game in the then soccer-crazed Seattle of the early 1980s. As youth soccer burgeoned, and as the ever more dazzling skill set of kids presented themselves at a younger and younger age, just who qualified for which team was fungible. In my case the real answer was whatever age Michael, a teenage soccer phenom, later with the Seattle Sounders soccer team, was. We adults claimed Michael as soon as our respective consciences would allow, and the teams were set from there.

Unwittingly on his part, man-child Michael exposed my loss of a step. On that memorable (if only to me) day, Michael, playing left wing, saw me, his counterpart on the right wing, streaking – at least in my mind toward the goal. Instinctively, he fired a perfectly located pass that initially eluded his and my defenders. The pass was exactly on target to where one of his usual teammates would have arrived at the precise time as the ball, assuring the teammate of a great shot on goal.

Despite herculean effort on my part to inject extra spring into my stride to be in the right place at the right time and do the right thing, the ball passed in front of my awkwardly extended right foot. At that moment in time, before God and all those witnesses, I had demonstrably lost a step.

Today, in my mind's eye I still see the angle of my foot as it struggled to contact the out-of-reach ball. Positioned in such a way that it could never have made solid contact with the ball, my foot had taken on the appearance of a limp, a disembodied appendage, that mockingly waved goodbye to my past physical prowess as I knew it, or, at least, had imagined it.

While saying goodbye that Fourth of July to vestiges of my youthful physical prowess, I sensed I no longer could forestall admitting psychological, spiritual, as well as physical realities; that, if ignored, would be perilous to my spiritual health, happiness and wholeness. The age-old question first encountered as a young adult – *What is the meaning of life?* Was now before me in 3-D. Such quandaries I had encountered at 20, were answered by conjecture. By middle age, such questions demanded answers along with matters of the spirit.

For me, as I suspect, for all at any age, the answers can be found in issues of identity. *Who am I? What do I identify with more closely, and on a personal level, with whom*? Such leading questions always beg for answers to further questions, such as *What roles do I play?* and *What is the quality of my relationships?*

Somewhere in this realm of personal interrogation lies the overtly spiritual question, *what is the role of a Supreme Being or Higher Power in my life?* For many, a relationship with such a being or power shapes one's identity. It gives meaning to life and drives its purpose and actions.

For the target audience of this book, whether 60 approaches or has passed, I have good news for you. Losing a step physically can adjust your focus so in future seasons you can see and embrace life's rich spiritual lessons of grace, perspective, patience, and acceptance. The gifts they bring allow us all to find the blessings that dwell in the depths of our spiritual nature. Embedded in these gifts might even be long-sought-after answers to life's thorny questions.

During our younger years, when we were more certain of our physical skills and mental acuity, we often took on an air of attacking projects and problems. We believed life needed to be conquered. In our latter years, head-to-head competition – inevitable, even necessary on many fronts at one time of our lives – no longer need preoccupy our time, efforts, and emotions. We need not see ourselves as either conquerors or the vanquished.

Cooperation, harmony, tranquillity, peacefulness, and serenity, a oneness, can become our new companions, filling our hearts with positive thoughts, freeing our minds to focus on important matters, saving our energy for living life fully, appreciating every day as never before. This can be a time we reach out to those we once viewed with suspicion, and even to perceived adversaries to discover they are friends, not foes.

Let me be clear; any newfound emphasis on the spiritual nature of what surrounds us need not and should not be at the expense of physical and mental focus and engagement. Take to heart everything the author says about the physical realities of this season and how to live with them. My plea is, as you stay active, make connections as to how your physical activities touch and enliven your spirit. Find the spiritual in the physical and mental arenas in your life.

This will bring you joy as you continue life-long pursuits, find renewed passion for long-ago abandoned activities, or engage in new ones. Whatever you do, push yourself. Walk that extra mile every morning and pray while you do so. Ski another year and give thanks for the Creation. Take a class about something you know absolutely nothing about and sense the wonder of continued learning. Do crossword puzzles in ink all the while patting yourself on the back for continued confidence and skill. Now is the time of life to discover fully the connective tissue that binds the physical, the mental, and the spiritual.

Much of our lives have been lived in the so-called Information Age. But information in isolation is limited. To reach its full potential for the benefit of humanity, information needs two companions – knowledge and wisdom. Knowledge gives shape, form, direction, and context to information. But wisdom is the real treasure in this trinity, for it brings a reflective quality and a perspective that nothing else can.

Past seasons have brought us experiences. If we have been alerted while gathering them, gaining wisdom has been the result. Wisdom's lessons can be counted as assets in our memory bank. We have paid the price for them. We own these experiences and these lessons free and clear. Enjoy them! Spend time with them, and (but only when asked!) share them. May those who spend time with you be wise enough to seek out your wisdom.

By 60, the issue of retirement is just that – an issue. Within your peer group you will know people who have retired, others who cannot wait to retire, and still others who refuse to think or talk about it. For some, "The R Word" or retirement itself seemingly surrounds all of life. It can become the unwanted elephant in the room of your life or your newfound best friend. But whatever your reality, you must deal with it.

As you do so, search for the spiritual potential it offers – it is present at every turn. At my 35th college reunion, which meant the attendees were in their mid-50s, I, along with an expert on technology and a physician, were part of a panel asked to address how we should be preparing for the future. Implicit in the focus was the issue of retirement.

At that time, retirement ages were more defined than today. Social Security and pension plan seemed ironclad. Baby Boomers and younger were employed to the hilt. The word gerontology was unknown to many. Retirement seemed to be an ill-defined nether land, a time of life after work ended, with the hope for a little leisure to be grabbed and good health bottled before death.

As a pastor, I have been fortunate to observe some for whom retirement was the fullest time of their lives, including spiritually. I have also witnessed self-defeating, even self-destructive post-retirement behaviours, that have led to misery, even death.

Accentuating the positive, I have observed that healthy retirees have some things in common. They plan for their retirement. They recognise that those 60 and above have more discretionary time than when they were younger, so they realise that time management is an issue. They seek a balance between being and doing, allotting healthy amounts of time for themselves and for others. They attend to matters of the spirit.

The happiest retirees I know are realistic about their resources of time, energy, physical condition, and finances. They recognise that there is no one right way to retire. They realise they might not "get retirement right" the first day off the job. Through trial and error and discernment, they find new or renewed purpose in life. They maintain a positive mental attitude. They find a daily, weekly, monthly, and annual rhythm that allows their lives to flow. They fill their spirits with what has meaning to them at this stage of their lives. How? They do not just retire in the typical sense of the word – they reinvest.

Successful retirees begin their reinvestment by embracing the opportunity to leave their decades-long occupation for new possibilities, activities, and relationships. They find new ways to self-identify. In this new season of their lives, they embody the concept of *carpe diem,* of seizing the day.

Healthy reinvestment can and should be both self-directed and other-directed. Self-direction begins with examining the interior of our soul and then feeding those cavities in our lives that hunger. The path to finding the essentials to making you feel whole begins with being alone, still, and silent. In her poem *Messenger,* the poet Mary Oliver points us to important elements for being in touch with ourselves and this season of our lives. *"Am I no longer young and still not half perfect? Let me keep my mind on what matters which is my work, which is mostly standing still and learning to be astonished."*

You may be yearning for intellectual stimulation or spiritual sustenance. In solitude, take time to heed the message of the X-shaped wooden train signs that caution motorists where train tracks cross a road. *Stop, Look, Listen.* Let the world around you do the talking; the enigmatic character in a book you are reading; a phrase from your religion's holy book; the squirrel or bird outside your window, or the picture on your living room wall you hung because of convention but, with concentrated looking, can speak the proverbial thousand words to you it never had before.

If you are prone to loneliness, by spending self-directed time in prayer, meditation, and reflection, you will be less lonely. Such time might even reintroduce you to someone you discover you really enjoy and wish to spend more time with – yourself! And as you feel a sense of wholeness within and about yourself, chances are others will want to spend time with you as well.

Other-directed activity is the logical response of those whose spiritual life is alive and robust. All the world's major religions tout service to others as part of their basic belief pattern. Reaching out is part of embracing all the created order and the creations that inhabit it. Those who do not reach out to others cheat both themselves and others. To be sure, the giving-receiving equation is not tit for tat. During some seasons of our lives, we give more than we receive. At other times, we are receivers more than givers.

Both moments, however, provide opportunities for grace given and received. This process allows our best selves and that of others to be revealed. This is where our holiness and the holiness of others can be revealed.

Meaningful, other-directed activity can be found in myriad places. The common thread is the opportunity for healthy interaction with others in some form of community. Faith communities that live up to the name – churches, synagogues, temples, mosques – can provide spiritual direction, intellectual stimulation and moral support while being a touchstone for helping us continually tapping into traditions that touch the core of our beings. Community centres and groups of every stripe allow healthy channels for the energies of those over 60. Seek out what you think will give your life meaning, purpose and energy – it will be the best investment you will ever make!

Those who believe in a creator whose nature is full of goodness seem to respond to life with an attitude of gratitude. What mobility is to physical health, gratitude is to spiritual well-being? Such a worldview lightens one's heart and puts a zip in one's clip. It renews (at least partially!) a spring in one's lost step. In the realm of cosmic math's equation of giving and receiving, an attitude of gratitude reveals this answer; no matter how much one gives, one always receives more in return.

Those who embrace an attitude of gratitude – who feel they can never pay back enough for all they have received – no matter to whom they attribute their good fortune, live spirit-filled lives. They feel rich in blessings, and they share their blessings, enjoying every opportunity to give. They are day-brighteners.

Remembering Ecclesiastes once more, we read of the contrasting activities of life's matters under heaven here on earth. While set forth as opposites, in terms of the life cycle, these matters are, in fact, complementary. Living finds its completion in dying. Crops planted in the spring demand harvesting in the fall. Acquiring knowledge, experiences, and possessions has its place, but finally wisdom and reflection are greater gifts.

Regarding possessions, in an age of storage units as a growth industry, the question we should be asking is *Do we possess our possessions, or do our possessions possess us?*

When the billionaire Howard Hughes died, someone asked, 'How much did he leave?'

Hearing the question, a wise onlooker answered, "Everything."

To comprehend fully the times life presents us, with their opposing actions and accompanying emotions, and to embrace these times with all our hearts, souls, minds and strength, our spirits must be open to the heights and depths life offers. Remember, we cannot understand laughter's healing properties until we have wept tears of anguish, despair and hurt. Likewise, the freeing exuberance that dance offers is best known only after something weighing us down has been a recent partner.

A way life-giving, spirit-filling events and opportunities waltz into our life and invite us to dance, is through rites, rituals, and ceremonies. Many observances that we name holy and celebrate today had their origins in ancient religious practices. Other practices sprung up because of creation's role in the human life cycle, often in relationship to the change of seasons. We observe days of national, local, or ethnic significance. Birthdays, weddings, anniversaries, funerals, reunions, and gatherings, inspired by countless events, take on celebratory and ritualistic qualities over time. These practices are part of what mark time and rites of passage. They are part of what makes us human.

These observances put us in touch with our past and those who have been part of it, and, at the same time, gives us hope for more of the good life has in store for us. However, the rites, rituals, and ceremonies that touch our lives originated and have become a part of your life – whether their origins were cultural, providential, or serendipitous. Name them, claim them, observe them, and share them, for they are a part of you. In many ways, they define you.

The truth is what we celebrate reflects what we value, even who we are. Remember; when the season arrives in which we are no longer physical beings, it is our spirit that will live on. In the meantime, in the spirit of thriving, not just surviving, I urge you to embrace the spiritual, as well as the physical, in all matters under heaven every day for the rest of your life.

Chapter 8
Invincibility Versus Invisibility

Over 60 invisibility overcomes the sense of vulnerability when we were younger. A bad headache becomes an imagined brain tumour. ER doctors react to a man over 60 with more affirmation than what is in a bag of medications. Society must dispel cultural myths real or perceived about an older man's vulnerability. Remember and quell not regret the exciting but often risky behaviour of our youth. Checking the obituaries in the Sunday paper is like checking the results from Monday night football – a man has won – if he has lived longer than most in this section of the paper. Men over 60, often invisible, are not always as vulnerable as society would believe they are. Dispel the mythology that we are a done deal.

"Some guy said to me: 'Don't you think you're too old to sing rock and roll?' I said, 'You'd better check with Mick Jagger.'"

– Cher, Actress

Freud's explanation of psychoanalysis as described by Didier Anzieu is a counter-phobic defence against anxiety through intellectualisation; permanently ruminating on the instinctive, emotional world that was the actual object of fear. I still prefer the inscription on an electric box near my home, "Think less, feel more."

About his cameo 85th birthday 10,000-foot parachute jump, President George H.W. Bush said, "Just because you are an old guy, you don't have to sit around drooling in the corner. Get out and do something. Get out and enjoy life."

"A Walk in The Woods" All Happened to Me

Everyone I know was terrified when I announced, 'I am going to do a "through" hike of the entire Superior Hiking Trail (SHT) alone.'

My eldest daughter screamed, 'No, Dad. No. Don't do it!'

Had she not been in LA, I am sure I might have set out on my journey with her arms tightly grasping my legs.

The SHT is a mere 310 miles stretching from Jay Cooke Park – 150 miles north of the Twin Cities – to Otter Lake Road, a few miles from the Canadian border. A "through" hike up and down countless streams and rivers running into Lake Superior stretches from Duluth to a Birdseye view of the Pidgeon River in the distance flowing through the Canadian Quetico Provincial Park. This is where the SHT connects with the Border Route Hiking trail. In length, the SHT is a mere freshman among the Great Trails. The Appalachian Trail (AT) stretches 2160 miles from Springer Mountain in Georgia to Katahdin, Maine. The Pacific Crest National Scenic trail, a long distance and equestrian trail closely aligned with the highest portion of the Cascade and Sierra Nevada Mountain ranges, runs 2,653 miles.

My bucket list trek began as I threw on what was an excessively heavy pack and taking a "selfie" in front of the entry point trail marker. It was only 10 minutes before I was having my first senior moment. I suddenly realised I was going south not north, my planned direction. Yeah, I get it, Lake Superior right, woods left. I would be in for plenty of surprises over the next month and a half. My pack always felt too heavy as it was weighted down with food for a week; an older heavy tent; clothes for every type of weather—let's call it," the hernia special". Late May into early June nights were so cold I could only stay warm if I wore ALL my clothes including my made-in-China rain suit that lasted less than a week before self-destructing.

I saw NO ONE for 60 miles. Trees had buds but no leaves. About the trail, vistas are awesome. There were no black flies yet. There were no mosquitos…. yet. There were no ticks…. yet. This early in the hiking season, all campsites are empty. Alone day after day early in the so early I the summer, there is just myself. I began hallucinating, imagining I was seeing signs of civilisation – houses, direction signs that, as I got closer, were in fact broken and bent trees or moss-covered boulders, dropped when the last ice age retreated

As spring was becoming summer, the mosquitos took their revenge. Luckily, this summer would not bring black flies. I savoured the silence and isolation. Meeting groups of loud hikers intruded on my Zen-like meditation.

As I hiked, with some days of constant rain. the weather and I went from dry to wet. Trees still had buds but no leaves. I knew I was often flirting with hypothermia. On another occasion and not blessed with the best sense of direction, I accidentally took a side trail and found myself doubling back, making several circles and feeling lost. I felt both frustrated and frightened.

On another occasion, while filtering water from a miniscule stream surrounded by boulders, I was attacked by mosquitos. I got up too fast for a 70-year-old man. I entered a twirling fall and slammed back against my pelvis. I was fortunate I missed hitting my head or hip. Alone and scores of miles from help, I was terrified and screamed. I feared I would not be able to walk. Yet, I was back on the trail the next day. I knew I had won a dance with serious injury and potential death.

I experienced excruciating pain on the side of my back over the largest bone of my pelvis where I had hit the boulder behind me. After a short time, I realised I had lucked out, and knew I had just bruised a pelvic bone and not a disc or a vertebra. For days I felt pain as I walked but that gradually left me.

The trail was blocked at one point, and I took a detour to the highway bordering the trail. As I was walking-in this case wrongly with the flow of traffic not toward it and deep in thought, I felt a rush of wind against the back of my legs. It was then that I realised that a car had almost hit me. The car that had swept by me was now in front of I me. Dirty, tired, and outright scared, it was then that I decided that there had to be a higher power looking after me. Such an entity had not been there to save me but, to warn me that if I kept doing stupid things I would die.

Beautiful vistas, wild rapids and falls, gorgeous maples, birches, cedars, and white or red pine were everywhere. The worst campsites were next to beaver ponds. Plenty of lodges but no beaver. Were they on vacation?. Huge moose prints were everywhere especially on the north part of the trail but, alas, I did not spot one. Were they visiting relatives? I did spot a few snowshoe rabbits who appeared to look at me sceptically. "Hey, pops, what's an old man like you walkin' around dees woods alone?" Just lucky, I guess.

I lived! When it was over, I was one proud 70-year old man. I had crossed another item off my bucket list. Mine became a walk on the wild side. I felt proud of an accomplishment that allowed me to relive the feeling of invincibility I had taken for granted before passing sixty. I proved to myself I still had the juice.

One Man's Shot to Sail Around the World

I met Kevin Holmes, the retired over-sixty draftsman and farmer from Durbin, South Africa while I was restoring a classic '62 Roamer Chris Craft on Lake Superior after my hike on the SHT. Over dinner aboard his new sailboat, I learned Kevin had already completed several around-the-world sails, but this time he was planning to do it solo. He explained that he flew from Durbin, bought a neglected forty-two-foot C&C birthed near my slip in this quiet sailing town of Bayfield, Wisconsin on Lake Superior. Over the next few weeks, I watched him make his boat seaworthy. I envied his anticipated over-sixty adventure.

"Isn't it terribly dangerous, Kevin, to go it alone across the ocean?' I asked one wiry, tough, and seasoned sailor as he danced effortlessly around the deck readying "The Pucho".

He carefully learned every inch of his compact craft. He knew that if he did not, he could die. Barefoot, he did pirouettes from winch to winch, halyard to halyard, checking and rechecking. Looking up to the blue sky, he checked the wind turbine on the mainmast He double checked the autopilot off the stern. Quiet and intense, he tested a mechanical winch off starboard.

"We are the instrument of our success," he explained.

The book he wrote about previous sailing adventures told me about his ongoing life fulfilling what other men shrug off as pipe dreams. He reassured me that he has circled the world by sailboat five times before assuring him he could go it alone. On his previous sails he had stopped for time to work in the Caribbean and later Australia. His planned route, he explained, would be through the Caribbean. Then he planned to sail from the infamous doldrums across to Brazil continuing his sail across the Equator and then through the "Roaring Forties" and on to Tristan da Cunha in the middle of the South Atlantic. "If all goes well," as Kevin explained, "I expect it will be free and clear around the Cape of Good Hope and back to my home in Durbin."

Planning and trying such a feat for Kevin or for any man our age, can be a last hoorah to challenge our invincibility. Powering by motor through the doldrums, in the Caribbean, Kevin unexpectedly ran out of kerosene that ran his bilge pumps. "The Pucho" sank. Kevin lived. Will he challenge his invincibility again? Some call behaviour like Kevin, Juho, and mine counter-phobic; not to fear the fear, as it were. let us call it an ongoing thirst for invincibility. Our risk taking can be an unconscious drive to challenge the angst, the fear that we can no longer take the kind of risk that was a way of our earlier life challenging imagined invincibility.

Flashback to College Days and Delusions of Invincibility

I still recall the moment Kip, my Dartmouth roommate and fellow adventurer, hit the median curb on a midweek road trip. Those tentative moments as the car rode the two wheels on the other side from the curb became a circus act complete with screams followed by laughter. We had defied gravity and avoided a near-death possibility by minimising our vulnerability.

On another occasion while mountain climbing, we were stalled on a granite ledge a thousand feet above the ground. We did not have enough rope to belay down, and the next climb to the top appeared too technical. The day was late, and we lacked enough equipment to bivouac on the ledge. This might have become a skirmish with hypothermia and even death—it snowed that night. We realized we could go neither up nor down. One of us had to climb ahead on belay from below, always significantly more dangerous, especially if a piton dislodges so the person climbing ahead goes into free fall. I took the challenge and climbed to the summit. Kip followed. Our risk-taking behaviour, based on imagined invincibility, were delusions that we had power and control of our environment. Another win for fictional invulnerability.

Freshman year at Dartmouth was more about achieving autonomy than about books and classes. My grades reflected my priorities. We considered ourselves invincible. For those of us over 60, perceptions of invincibility are tempered by reality. I spoke about the value of age-adjusted decisions in the chapters on "Cognition" and "Balance and Gait" as an important way to avoid the accidents such as the ones I may not have survived. Age-related changes to proprioception, vision, and the vestibular function over 60, needs be reckoned with. I emphasise that we should think before plunging forward when there is a greater risk of an accident.

Widespread belief held by society is that we should no longer live life on the edge. Why not? What do we have to lose? But, what do we hear? "Slow down!" But why? There is still fun to be had. I do sometimes fail to heed such warnings. Certainly, go at it with a dose of discernment. There are realistic considerations about age-related cardiac risks; or, more brittle bone that add into the liability equation. "Beware!" naysayers warn. The earlier seasons of our lives described by sociologist, Daniel Levinson in *The Seasons of a Man's Life*, confirm how our fast our years have shot by-too fast at that.

Alas, we have hurtled through pre-adulthood, early adulthood, middle adulthood, and have; at last, and hopefully gone not kicking or screaming, arrived at late adulthood (60–85). We may be blind-sided by the reality that we are ageing – I hope gracefully. High school and college years slid into early and middle adulthood. As we rambled through many rites of passage, we immersed ourselves in solid relationships, children, and demanding early and late careers. Now, the task is visualising vulnerability but, at the same time, not becoming preoccupied by it but, courageously, moving into our retirement years. We still have opportunities to challenge ourselves and our environment but now, consider tempering the impulse with realistic expectations.

Our skills behind the wheel change over the years. Bravado and daring do combine with acting-out behaviour that may often be reckless, explaining the high insurance rates for teenagers. Ageing brings cataracts, declining night vision, slower reflexes, and challenges performing complex movements with our earlier alacrity. As elders, we learn to compensate. In an earlier chapter I describe how concert musicians must practice more to maintain their craft.

Ageing drivers just must become more cautious. The hell with going over 85 unless you are living in LA. Every time I drive up on a slow car in the right lane with the driver hunched low behind the wheel, head forward, both hands clenched on the wheel, I know it is an oldster and suspect the time has come for him or her to make an appointment at the department of motor vehicles testing centre. That should include a vision and hearing screen.

Different from our invincible selves of late adolescence, we are less likely to take risks – or so car insurance statistics confirm. We must compensate for the later decline in mechanical and sensory skill. Despite all such cautions, by the time we hit 80, the chance of a motor vehicular accident is five times greater than for the younger driver.

An octogenarian has a three times greater chance of dying in an automobile accident. The medications that our doctor prescribe, sometimes inadvisably, can slow our response time and also contribute to an accident or death. My advice: watch out for the cops because one slipup and you may get pulled over for a DWO, driving while old. Recently, I was stopped by a police officer near my home: "Hey, you are only a few blocks from home," he says. I know that's in my favour. He knows from my license I am over 75. "Do you know what the speed limit is, sir?" "Fifty-five, officer." "Try 35, sir!." You know you are old (er) when someone, in this case a police officer at your window, addresses you as "Sir." "I thought I was going with the flow of traffic, officer." His response is not favourable. "Are you kidding me, you do know how fast you were going?" Again; "I know now, officer.": Important: be polite before you start begging. You know he is also checking out your age and, based on your age, is checking out if you are working with a full deck. In your favour, you are a senior and not a teenager. Good time for begging now. "Please, officer, I hope you are not going to give me a ticket." Silence. Another glance at the driver's license. "That picture of you, sir, is really strange." "Yes," I answer. "They told me to open my eyes and my lids really have gotten droopy." Humour can sometimes be helpful as I play on the vicissitudes of ageing; in this case, drooping lids.

We are supposed to be "risk-avoidant" over 60. But what happened to me? Once again, I advise moderation in moderation. Sure, keep taking risks. Think first, and, realistically, act second.

Chapter 9
Sex Is Not a Dirty Word Over 60

Despite what society thinks about our sexual vitality, men over 60 crave shared physical intimacy and love. Listen to your inner voice how sexuality works for you and can be equally shared. A 40-year marriage may not preclude a shift to homosexuality – a great number of gay men are married. Turn-ons for men change. Cues shared, regardless of sexual orientation, bear more similarities than differences. Direct touch now surpasses visual cues. Bring tenderness, innovation, and; above all, communication to the bedroom. Pillow talk, nonsexual touching, and sweet words are aphrodisiacs. Women lose partners or have physical changes such as vaginal dryness. Men often have old sports or work injuries that can make weight bearing painful thus calling for adaptation of sexual positions rather than abstention. Erectile dysfunction is treatable. Sex is safe and ageless. Yet, those of us over 60 are equally susceptible to STDs as those younger. There can be sex after prostatectomy and, may even be better following joint replacement. Stay fit. Eat right. Strive for a positive view of life past 60 and expect to enjoy sex into your 80s. Sexuality is a powerful affirmation of life refusing to give in to death.

"Life without sex might be safer but it would be unbearably dull."
– H.L. Mencken, Writer

This chapter is about sex for men over sixty and how to continue or renew its enjoyment. You're wondering where I'm going with that. I realised (finally!) that I was writing this chapter from a heterocentric perspective. In the process I realised ignoring a significant percentage of our population, gay and bisexual, was insulting to my gay friends who deserve inclusivity rather than exclusivity.

The estimate of the male gay population may be 6% and, most likely, underestimated based on a gay or bisexual man over 60 fearing exposure; or in some level of denial. That a man might admit he is attracted sexually to men may only surface later in life and surprise everyone close, especially his wife. A soft figure is that 40% of gay or bisexual men are married – many of whom have children – and unquestionably and deservedly are good fathers.

I realised I knew little about gay sex among older men my age and did a long-overdue education about a different orientation from my own that I knew little about. There is a saying, "There are greater differences within groups than between them." Surprisingly, I discovered that, instead of differences regarding sexuality between gay and non-gay men our age, that there are many similarities between both groups about sex and relationships.

A significant percentage of gay men over 60 share feelings of loneliness or "wistful" yearning just as among men who are straight. Random sex takes the same emotional toll for either men who have sex with men (MSM) or men who have sex with women(MSW):that of emptiness and lack of fulfilment. As Robin Bell describes, both cultures over 60 may finally step off "The unconscious and relentless treadmill of desire." When I reflect on men over 60 in heterosexual or same sex relationships, a bad relationship or marriage of either can be equally unfulfilling.

Men over 60, gay or straight, who choose to have multiple partners are equally at risk for STDs. Internet dating has revolutionised all relationships and hook ups. Gone are a significant amount of the destructive behaviours such as anonymous sex associated with pre-epidemic HIV. Two-thirds of gay men have anal sex occasionally. Ten % do so regularly. Unprotected, this practice increases the risk of HIV; whereas, vaginal penetration in MSW is the same as for other STDs. Fortunately, we now have PrEp (oral pre-exposure prophylaxis) that is 99% effective preventing sexually transmitted or 74 % effective against injection caused HIV.

Gay or straight, we live in a society centred around youth and beauty. Such youth orientation has been especially identified with much of the gay culture. Sex of either heterosexual or same sex relationship in our prime is described as equally protean although the intensity begins to wane past 60. The better news is that we are now mature and, hopefully wiser. The straight world has many misconceptions about gay men. A goodly percentage of gay men have many of the same challenges of heterosexual men over 60. Sexual dysfunction affects men of all sexual preferences.

Just as with straight couples, whoever is on top or the bottom during intercourse, does not define either role as active versus passive. If the man or woman is on the bottom, they are still the man or woman, respectively. Consensual anal penetration requires as much preparation and understanding as vaginal sex. Good sex for either gay or straight men requires compassion, creativity, patience, don't forget, communication.

Applicable to gays and straights alike is that men over 60 are no longer as easily aroused by visual stimuli as when we were younger. At this benchmark age, men usually take longer to become aroused. Past 60, arousal is more neurogenic; sensory nerves respond more to affectionate caresses and oral stimulation. We are also not necessarily getting better, but taking longer.

Sex in older couples is a shared endeavour. A partner who has aged with you may now experience declining estrogen and progesterone or, if in a male-male relationship, testosterone. A woman in perimenopause experiencing atrophy of the mucous secreting cells lining the vagina, has less hormonally derived lubrication that enhanced earlier mutual pleasure. A woman, also – especially after a period of limited sexual activity-may develop vaginal narrowing called stenosis, making intercourse painful or impossible without adequate lubrication or, if indicated and desired, physician guided dilation.

Anal and vaginal sex can require patience and must be consensual especially involving a man with a large penis or a woman with a less compliant vagina. Men who choose anal sex should have some water-based lubricant ready beforehand that will not destroy a condom or sexual intensity. Patience is of the essence either with ongoing, renewed, new vaginal, or anal sex. Gay men have no greater incidence of piles or rectal fissures. Heterosexuals are in search of the illusive g-spot just as gays explore for the prostate spot. Preferences for gays is oral sex, genital to genital, mutual masturbation, and anal penetration.

Unprotected anal sex risks exposure to Giardia and hepatitis B or C. Gays or straights with multiple partners change the playing field. Men having sex with men (MSM) are at risk for STDs from oral, anal, and rubbing skin to skin (frottage). HIV, Chlamydia, and gonorrhoea are spread through sexual fluids such as semen and other body fluids. HIV and hepatitis B are spread by blood, contaminated needles, and unprotected sex. Genital herpes, syphilis, and human papillomavirus (HPV) may be spread through genital or skin-to-skin contact. STDs have no sexual preference. Hepatitis B and C, as well as HIV, can be prevented by careful initial sexual activity avoiding body secretions or blood using condoms or dental dams until infection of either partner is ruled out. Sexually transmitted human papilloma virus (HPV) from oral sex is associated with throat cancers.

There are egregious misconceptions about differences between those of us who prefer women and those who enjoy men. Sexologist, Robin Bell, in the *British Medical Journal*, extols how anarchic gay humour sustains gay men. None of us over 60 have volunteered to join the older set. But, today's 60s are yesterday's 50s. What gay and straight men have in common is exploring how our sex lives can now be more zestful and, in fact, become the best we have known. Sexual function changes. We have less frequent spontaneous erections. We experience diminished engorgement. We experience longer refractory period between orgasms – if we are fortunate to have more than one. Forty percent of men over 50 – gay or straight, experience some sexual challenges of which two-thirds are physiological.

Keeping hydrated is extremely important for lubrication. Drink plenty of water and natural juices. Hydration is the simplest first and best way to improve secretions. That means water not coffee. Caffeine is a diuretic and dries scetions. Antihistamines, tricyclic anti-depressants, atypical antipsychotics, and cancer medications also can dry us out.

Women in a heterosexual relationship have a much greater chance of losing a sex partner. Men die earlier. One older woman friend confided, "My husband dropped dead on the tennis court. I told him to stick to doubles"! Men and women have different reasons why they change their sexual activity. An ageing male partner may experience physical limitations such as bad knees or lower back arthritis. Consequently, we may no longer engage in the form of sex we enjoyed over a lifetime and that worked so well over the past decades. An older man in a healthy gay relationship, similarly and often more with a younger partner, can experience identical challenges. An open attitude between both partners is laden as much with surprise as necessity.

A woman's or widowed older gay man's sexual possibilities has more to do with having a willing, available, and able partner. Judy Moore LMFT, a noted Davis, California family and marriage therapist, tells us that ageing women can become invisible and, understandably, are less likely to have an opportunity for sex. Why should such a predicament be different for an over 60 gay man? But, interest in sex persists. For a widowed woman or gay man, sexual activity appears to be driven by accessibility. HIV decimated a gay culture that thrived on anonymous multi-partner, and often illicit sex relegated to bathrooms, bars, bathhouses, or back alleys. The internet has changed the playing field for gays and straight men and women alike by providing less person-to-person immediate contact with better screening for a safer and hopefully, ultimately dynamite hook up.

Maintaining a satisfying mutual sex life as we age – especially in a long-term relationship – requires being less self-centred with a willingness to explore innovative techniques that can create a loving and mutual gratification. Make a date for nonsexual intimacy. Validate with words and non-sexual cuddling how important a seasoned lover continues to be for you. Don't be afraid to tell your partner how much you love him or her. A relationship always needs the feeling of closeness, tenderness, and communication.

Sadly, certain male-dominated cultures ignore the vital importance of another man or woman's arousal and pleasure. Such self-focus does not know sexual preference. Holding, cuddling, gentle words, and mutual, non-sexual touching are wonderful foreplay for the best way to begin wonderful sex. If you want sex to be great, keep it mutual. Both partners need to feel safe expressing what either likes or dislikes. What better way to ensure an encore the next week, or sooner. Lean back and enjoy.

The preferences for satisfaction for gay men and a non-gay alike are intimate kissing, oral sex, mutual masturbation, genital-to-genital contact, or anal sex – euphemistically called "Vanilla" sex by my gay friend. Three-fourths of gay men say they are content with their sex lives. The intensity and variation for MSM and MSW are not necessarily apples and oranges. The missionary or standing cowgirl positions are not hetero-patented. During sex play, either partner can do a flip-flop, trading places.

Sexual intensity does not plummet with the length of a relationship. Robin Bell in The *British Medical Journal* (1999), describes how maturity can replace "the unconscious, relentless mechanical treadmill of desire.". Among straights and gays, sexual activity is enhanced by several factors. By this later chapter in our lives, we know and more easily express what turns us on. We are less self-conscious. We may be less engaged in work-our children are well on their way, and we have more free time–no more time clock to worry about. We can shift from the focus of an immediate orgasm to a fuller erotic and sensual life. Cuddling as well as emotional closeness always ranks first.

To ensure our own sexual gratification earlier in our lives, we may have been more selfish. Maybe, we just didn't know how to satisfy a woman or another man. In a testosterone storm, we were less concerned if our partner was genuinely enjoying sex, but often more concerned of our own getting off. Mutual gratification was not always a priority. There comes a day of cruel awakening when the proud angle of our erection no longer aims for the sky and, worse yet, may now be flying at half-mast. The welcoming news is that after 60, our machinery is still workable and sustainable. Our sex lives can benefit from creativity, understanding, and, above all else, communication. But I risk being repetitive.

A superior relationship of any sexual orientation requires respect and tenderness. In long-term relationships, what worked earlier to enhance each other's sexual pleasure may no longer be a turn-on. Sexual disharmony may not be the reason for a failing sexual relationship, but the result of turmoil in our relationship. Major arguments between couples about sex and money can easily sabotage intimacy. Deeper personal struggles such as losing self-esteem and value after retirement accompanied by depression may better explain why things are not going great in bed. Retarded ejaculation, inability to achieve or maintain an erection, is as much from emotional stressors as from physical causes.

Once you both have honestly cleared the air of any ongoing problems, there is an opportunity on a date over a candlelit dinner, to explore easy-to-remedy delicate subjects as to how to improve each other's sexual pleasure. An older man or woman's body or mind issues – painful knees, a bad back, or emotional setbacks – if not honestly discussed, can threaten mutual pleasuring. Degenerative joint disease from work or sports-related problems can prevent weight bearing and disqualify an older man from enjoying active pleasurable sex. It is time now, to think out of the box, Ingenuity may be the mother both of invention, and a passport to new-found sexual pleasure.

I want to dispel some sexual myths among male-male relationships as different from the heterosexual preference. Three quarters of gay men report that they are content with their sex lives. Does this statistic apply to MSW? More than one half of gay men interviewed say they have sex once a week "in addition to the masturbating most men do". Do you mean OTHER men beat off? Whatever your sexual inclination, the key words are still communication, compassion, creativity, and patience to enhance our sex lives in our later decades.

First, let's get it straight (pun) that regardless of sexual preference, creative positions can enhance our sexual enjoyment. The missionary position may well have served both partners for decades. Physical limitations such as swollen painful knees or a crumbling back, can make this tried-and-true position painful. I encourage consulting books or videos that can enlighten you and your partner of alternative positions you both may never have considered but that now can bring unimaginable surprises.

Misconceptions abound about gay sex. Most positions described are easily applicable to gays and straights alike. Two-thirds of gay men practice penetrative anal sex on a regular basis. British studies among a younger cohort report that heterosexual women have a similar percentage of anal sex as gays. Describing the partner in whatever sexual orientation as the active and passive partner is way out of style. The Center for Disease Control and Prevention has found nearly the exact same percentages of anal sex for both men and women.

Now, for a few attainable options. Consummating desires with your woman or man sitting on top of you, facing forward, called the Cowboy or backwards, as the Reverse Cowboy, is not a sexual activity you will learn about in your orthopaedist's office after knee or back surgery. The latter position offers a way to fondle your lover's breasts while kissing the back of her/his neck or back searching for previously undiscovered and surprisingly sensitive places.

Keep an open mind that any new position can be another open expression of love and fun. I have not heard of a man turning down so pleasurable form of sexual expression as a lap dance. Don't be afraid to ask what turns your lover on. The catalyst for mutual pleasure can lie in something so simple as good communication. Prepare to listen. Let your lover coach you. Your partner knows their body better than you do. Ageing and familiarity can modify and improve time-tested sexual satisfaction.

The feminist movement heralded by books like *Our Body Ourselves*, by the Boston Women's Health Book Collective, changed many of the expectations held by both sexes. The tidal wave that empowered women also validated womanliness and the right to sexual satisfaction. Betty Freidan in *The Feminine Mystique* said it well, "Men are not the enemy, but the fellow victims. The real enemy is women's denigration of themselves."

It is time to get down to specifics. A woman's clitoris is an object of pleasure worthy of veneration. So too is the head of our penis. The next vital ingredient for rewarding sex is learning how to unselfishly turn on our partner. Pleasuring your lover brings shared joy for both of you. John Gray's *Men are from Mars, Women Are from Venus* emphasises how men and women think and feel differently. Based on our communication and awareness of selfless sexuality, many men have only managed to reach Pluto.

A man's orgasm is often shorter than that of a woman. Arousal for good sex to happen is less visual for women and more dependent on warming verbal cues as well as non-sexual touch. Women may take longer for arousal and to achieve orgasm. This pattern may change for a man over 60. A man's challenge is more often premature orgasm or erectile dysfunction (ED). The male orgasm is a complex system involving multiple hormones and nerve pathways. In the fifties Alfred Kinsey described the orgasm as an "explosive discharge of neuromuscular tension."

Arteriosclerotic vascular disease, calcifications, and diminished elasticity of smaller arteries may compromise those in the penis just as with coronary and cerebral vessels. Such changes affect blood vessels that enhance blood flow to the penis that are responsible for engorgement and an erection staying hard. These physical changes often combined with emotional issues can lead to ED.

In the eighties, research from the Sexual Awareness Research (SAR) Centre at the University of Minnesota Medical School, described a male orgasm as type I, a series of six to 15 regular pelvic muscle contractions over 20–30 seconds that is similar for both men and women. A type II orgasm, especially in women, lasts longer. Women can enjoy multiple orgasms each lasting an average of 13–51 seconds. Twenty-five percent of women fail to experience an orgasm from vaginal intercourse. Genital stimulation, deep kissing, and oral sex can be the golden trio for a man or woman to reach orgasm. Just take in any Netflix miniseries for the myth that would have us believe that both partners reach a simultaneous orgasm after immediate penetration frequently standing up.

Women can fake orgasm. Just watching and listening to Meg Ryan at lunch with Billy Crystal in *When Harry Met Sally* fake an orgasm over coffee should dispel any illusions we have about the fidelity of a woman's orgasm or that we are responsible for it. Such a male illusion belongs on the fiction shelf. You can ask your lover what lifts the curtain for the first act. Billy Crystal had his ah-ha moment. Reality bite: your penis is not necessarily what makes a woman or another man climax.

Stimulation of the clitoris or glans penis produces intense sexual pleasure. Seventy to 80% of women require direct manual or oral clitoral stimulation to reach orgasm. The outer third of the vagina contains nearly 90% of the vaginal nerve endings. The area around the labia minora and the urethra are also very sensitive. Just as female hormones decline past menopause, so does testosterone for ageing men. Our lubricating juices diminish as does that of our partner's natural lubricants. Men over 60 may have a decreased seminal fluid but sperm may still be viable.

Postmenopausal women can have an increased sexual interest and desire. Word of caution; just because we are over sixty does not mean we cannot get a 55-year-old woman pregnant especially if she is in menopause. Irregular menstruation during perimenopause increases the pregnancy risk. During this period of hormonal limbo, condoms, a spermicide, mutual masturbation, or oral sex are a pleasurable and safer alternatives to unprotected intercourse.

At last, an empty nest can bring unexpected joy and the opportunity to enjoy more uninhibited sex. With the children departed and that you are no longer chained to an eight-hour job, why not have some fun? "Let's do it on the upper landing." "No, we did that yesterday. Let's do it on the kitchen table!" Your penis may surprise you and become alive and hard again. If not, oh well, we will get to that later. There is a misconception that, when we are over 60, much of our sexual appetite resides above the shoulders rather than below the belt. By that I mean thinking about it but not doing it. Thinking negatively can sabotage opportunity.

We CAN continue sex into our eighties. Advertisements on TV extol Cialis and Viagra. Is ED an epidemic? Some of the guys in these advertisements look younger than us. Certainly, their partners do. Are erection aides where society is going?

Early in arousal, the carrier fluids in men over 60 from Cowper's glands diminish. Consequentially, the quantity of our ejaculate diminishes. Do not fret, orgasm is delightful despite the decrease or absence of the love juice of our youth. We may ask, "Hey, isn't your fantasy working either?" Failure breeds failure. Now we are getting into the "head" thing. Men may experience erectile dysfunction (ED) ranging from an inability to get and sustain an erection to premature ejaculation. Insecurity because of an unexpected loss of an erection does not signal the end of your sexual career. Plenty of medications ranging from the SSRIs like Prozac (fluoxetine), antihistamines like Benadryl (diphenhydramine), or a benzodiazepine like Xanax (alprazolam) notoriously may contribute to ED.

ED is no stranger to cinema. "Painless Pole" Waldowski, humorously known as "The best equipped dentist in the Army," and "The Dental Don Juan of Detroit", in the original *Mash*, becomes maudlin after experiencing a sexual misadventure and doubts his potency. To the strains of Mike Altman's *Suicide is Painless,* he elects for assisted suicide with The Black Pill. Robert De Niro in *Dirty Grandpa* graphically humanises the sexual frustrations of men over 60 especially when widowed. He is elated with a new lease on sex. "I just want to get laid," and, as a denouement, he has a baby with his significantly younger paramour.

Ageing past 60 does not spell the end of sexual pleasure. Although in our sixties and seventies our bodies and sexual responses are evolving, and our bodies may not always work in the accustomed way. Society often fails to understand that grandpa can have sex over sixty. Just as overcoming stereotypes applies to so many areas of our persona, so too, does sexuality. We may take longer for arousal and may require more stimulation. Creativity can enhance how we show love. Our goal is not only mutual gratification but a way we can express our love. Cher Winston, in *Woman's Anatomy: Secret Maps to Buried Treasure,* speaks for keeping sexual energy alive.

Betty Dodson, the well-known sex therapist, and author of *The Orgasm Doctor,* debunks societal mythology. "Many believe that sex for old people is non-existent, disgusting, or downright laughable." Joan Price, in *Naked at Our Age*, and an advocate for ageless sexuality, writes, "American Seniors… are extremely interested in sustaining sexual activity." In this potentially challenging final third of our lives, it is an opportune time NOT to say nay to sex.

My children become unsettled when I honestly admit I still have sex. I had the same shock at 21 when my father confided that he and my mother were still sexually active. My father was paraplegic from polio since he was thirty-three. His admission confirms that, even with a disability, an individual over sixty can and should desire the sexual tenderness of a loving relationship as my late and always prescient father had maintained with my mother.

My advice is to stay physically active, fit, find a willing partner, and – if it is your spouse of half a century – be creative, lean back, and enjoy, enjoy, enjoy. Erection or no erection, there are many ways to thread the needle. I wrote this chapter when I was celibate for over two years. Surprisingly, this is the longest chapter in the book. During the two years after my divorce, I limit expectations primarily for finding a willing partner not for sex, l companionship for a weekly concert. My electronic search was disapp When I least expected it, I fell into a full and reciprocal loving relationship with a younger woman – 19 years but who's counting. How sweet it is.

Dodson notes, "A hardy sexual and loving relationship can be a thrust for life again. It is said that sexuality represents the most powerful affirmation in the face of death." A man of 60 or older while brushing his teeth, may gaze into the bathroom mirror to be greeted by sagging and wrinkled skin. He may ask, "Is that me?" Non-judgmental acceptance of a loving partner has no equal.

Dodson advises that a man can exclaim, "My best teacher is my wife who tells me, "I love your body," or "You are the handsomest man in my world." "No, no," you may exclaim, "My stomach is not flat like when we first dated." How wonderful this may feel if our lover's reassurance is, "You look so good to me just the way you are."

Dodson further explains, "Masturbation is the foundation for all human sexuality. Our infants unconsciously do it. Married, and unmarried men, and women do it." Bergstrom and his co-authors report that men from sixty to eighty masturbate at least once a month." I got them beat if you will excuse the pun. So, why guilt yourself doing what most men our age do? Mark Hanna (Matthew McConaughey) in *The Wolf of Wall Street,* asks Jordon Belfort (Leonardo DiCaprio), "How many times a day do you beat off?" Most men of all ages masturbate as long as they live. There are those who unabashedly admit they do so… and those that lie.

An honest affirmation of feeling may well reverse a lifetime pattern of self-centeredness. Emotional intimacy applies to both genders. Sexuality is not just about you. It is also about our partner. Its joy requires a mutual feeling of safety. Why did it have to it take a quarter of a century for me to appreciate mutual satisfaction? It is never too late to discover a pleasurable closeness toward our lover.

Once we entered a room with an erection in front of us. Now, it is behind us. On a college first date, we made bedtime plans before the barista finished making the latté. As an elder we make our moves more slowly, building up to the pleasure for a new lover, or seducing our partner of 30 years. Blood flow to an ageing penis or our partner's vagina and clitoris may well have become slower. An ageing man takes more time for arousal and to achieve an orgasm. Pepper Schwartz, AARP's Love and Relationship Ambassador, reports that 50% of respondents use a sex toy to enhance sex.

The vibrator has been around since the 19th century. Assisting love making with one is not a crutch. There is no reason to think vibrators are kinky but rather that they can enhance sexual pleasure. There are many ways to build up to an erection and orgasm by stimulating the head of the penis or clitoris with a vibrator. One study reports that around 50% of respondents enjoy one.

Introducing a vibrator into lovemaking should be based on the agreement between two partners about "inviting" a vibrator into the bedroom. A vibrator is not a third person with you two in bed. There are many types and cost of vibrators including a bunny vibrator for your woman that can pleasure both the clitoris and the outer third of the vagina, the two most sensitive parts of a woman's vagina. There's plenty of options as well for older gay guys. A vibrator tells no tales and can help create and sustain arousal and enhance orgasm.

The common question that is often raised is, "Can I have sex again after my total prostatectomy (TURP)?" The answer is a resounding "Yes!" A radical prostatectomy, the removal of the entire prostate surrounding the urethra in more extensive cancer, can affect an erection and orgasm. However, it does not need to spell the end of erections or orgasm indefinitely. After prostatectomy, a man may not have an erection for up to a year or may take as long as two years. After such surgery he may experience retrograde ejaculation backwards into the bladder.

Robotic surgery can spare nerves important for orgasm. After surgery and removal of the seminal glands a man will no longer have the secretions associated with an orgasm. Also, pelvic floor muscles leading to the tension and anticipation of orgasm may be injured in surgery. After the operation and in recovery there are alternative ways for a man to share sexual gratification with their partner with a vibrator, manually, or with oral sex.

Sometimes it is a tough sell to men that an erection does not define manliness. If medications such as Viagra or Cialis fail to enhance an erection, due to distracting emotions, or, simply, from ageing, injections of alprostadil into the penis has 80% effectiveness. A penile urethral suppository, half the size of a grain of rice called MUSE(prostaglandin E1), inserted into the penis can be 30 to 40% effective. Another option is an implanted semi-rigid or inflatable plastic prosthesis.

Good sex should be about taking turns. Doctor Ruth in *Dr Ruth's Encyclopaedia of Sex* or her *Sex for Dummies* advises seniors that they should not be afraid to explore out of the box sex that is innovative but should have mutual acceptance. Sexual enjoyment means taking turns. Communicating carefully, while sharing previously unspoken needs, is vital to avoid frightening our partner.

In *Great Sexual Positions for Menopausal Women,* Madeline Vann, MPH, advocates that our partner can try changing the game, as it were, by try being on top or bottom during sex. This route to pleasure allows someone to control the position, pressure, and pace of intercourse. By doing so, our partner finds the best position to stimulate the clitoris or prostate and experience comfortable penetration. Being on top may be more comfortable should your partner have insufficient moisture or there is a size challenge. This is the time for plenty of pillows to knees, back, and elbows improving contact with erogenous zones.

It is fun to have your woman (or man) straddling you either facing forward or backward while you are sitting comfortably. This is a knee-friendly position. Our partner can kneel on pillows or stand on the floor next to the bed while our partner can lie comfortably on pillows bent over the edge of the bed. Ruth Westheimer in *Sex After 50: Revving up the Romance, Passion & Excitement!*

(Quill Driver Books 2005), offers a comprehensive over-view of pleasurable positions. Lisa Sweet's *365 Sex Positions: A New Way Every Day for a Steamy, Erotic Year!* is packed with realistic and exciting erotic positions.

A disabled man or woman with a physical challenge such as a spinal cord injury, can unabashedly enjoy sex with the modestly priced Intimate Rider. Once again, communication between partners can overcome otherwise insurmountable barriers.

Jose A. Rodguez, M.D. reports that 80% of 132 men reported improved and more frequent sex after joint replacement. In a recent study, 90% of participants report an improved sex life after hip or total knee surgery. Marty Kline, a Palo Alto sex therapist, confirms AARP's message. "Making love may be just the medicine you need to resolve joint pain. Everything about sex, can be good. It is terrific for people. Sex provides gentle range of motion stretching joints and muscles." Better sex improves overall well-being and self-esteem.

Sex can minimise pain and inflammation. Making love releases natural endorphins in the same fashion as enjoying special foods, massage, or just enjoyable and happy times. There is no shame in getting therapy. The Society for Sex Therapy and Research, The American Board of Sexology, The American Association of Sexuality, Educators, Counsellors, and Therapists, and The Society for Sex Therapy, are great resources to find a therapist who can assist an older man's journey to better sex. Asking for assistance can help rediscover your relationship and love life.

Cardiac issues, if compromised, can affect the flow of blood to the penis and vagina affecting arousal and lubrication. The physiological changes of hypertension, diabetes, and depression need not aversely effect having good sex. Open heart surgery takes time to heal, and a man and his partner may have reservations about resuming sex after surgery. Dr Joanne Foody, director of Cardiovascular Wellness Services at Harvard-affiliated Brigham and Women's Hospital, notes, "Heart attacks rarely occur during sex." Less than five % of anginal attacks are attributable to sexual activity... so-called 'angina d' amour'.

There are a host of medical challenges that need not interfere with sex. A temporary or permanent colostomy with a stoma is no reason to avoid love making. Your partner need take special care engaging in sex if you are immunosuppressed. Alternative techniques and considerations can allow sharing not abandoning our lover. Emotions and feelings for a partner can make sex adaptive and joyous.

Sex advisors remind us that the TV or, of late, other electronic devices like our laptop. Cell phone, or iPad, belong more in the living room than the bedroom. Watching tasteful, sensual, and woman and man-friendly videos hitherto called "porn" may be helpful if both of you agree. Responsible pornography can be a way to get the love juices flowing. Enjoyment should be mutual and that they have been made respectfully for the actors.

Arousal is slower as we age, and men can be unable to attain or sustain an erection. The penis or cock ring is just a shelf down from the condoms at your pharmacy or in a fantasy sex store. Safety and quality are imperative. A cock or tension ring can sustain the blood supply in an erect penis. A man must remove the ring immediately after orgasm to empty the engorged blood vessels in the penis. Incidentally, if you find the "G Spot" let me know. Then there is the "P" spot, which, reputedly, can be ignited with deliberate arousal during anal sex.

Ben WA, Burmese, Venus, or Geisha balls can be painlessly and consensually inserted into your lover's vagina or anus or yours as well to stimulate the pubococcygeus muscles that may improve orgasm. Take care inserting objects into the anus. Some objects may be difficult to retrieve. Butt plugs or anal beads may well be a turn on but must be safely tethered. Rectal intercourse is fine if consensual but, insertion depends on suitable lubrication to avoid pain. Slow and gentle is foremost.

Lubrication enhances successful intimacy especially if your partner has vaginal dryness, has developed vaginal stenosis, or has an anal fissure. There are plenty of pleasurable options.

- A silicone-based lubricant like Astrolide is plastic sex toy, condom-friendly, vegetable-derived, water-based, paraben free, sweet tasting, non-staining, and inexpensive. If mutually agreeable, it works well for anal sex. They cause less irritation and last longer than other lubricants. It is easy to find in the pharmacy and also shelved next to the condoms. This lubricant is water-friendly and can be great for sex in a lake, pool, or the hot tub. Take care, however, to avoid an infection from unsafe water.
- Oil-based lubricants are not latex condom friendly, but safely used with natural condoms.
- Polyunsaturated and plant-based natural oils like avocado, peanut, grapeseed, apricot, or olive oil are right on the kitchen shelf. If safe to eat, they are also safe for vaginal, anal, or oral sex.
- Petroleum-based lubricants like Vaseline, body lotions, and skin creams are fine for masturbation for both men and women, but stain, destroy condoms, and may prove irritating.

Using a condom is not just for teenagers. Men over 60 who are sexually active into their 80s, are still at risk for STD's – Chlamydia, both specific, gonorrhoea, ("GC" or "The Clap"), or nonspecific urethritis, syphilis and HIV-with unprotected sex. STDs are of equal concern to those over 60 as they are for younger men. They can be extremely uncomfortable and one, HIV, if untreated, has lethal consequences. Although all STDs can be treated, they can be painful and a hassle. STDs are passed by oral, anal, and skin-to-skin sex.

Summing up the often ignored topic of sexual fulfilment for men over 60, family, friends, and society should not deny that a man past sixty can continue to have a natural and sustained sexual appetite. Joan Price, author of *Naked at Our Age: Talking Out Loud About Senior Sex,* and *The Ultimate Guide to Sex after 50,* describes herself as a "self-styled advocate for ageless sexuality." She advocates a spicey satisfying sex Life that men and women over sixty deserve.

Attention to exercise, diet, mental health, communication, and creativity are essential for gratifying physical and emotional sexuality.

That society fails to accept that a man over sixty can desire and, more importantly, is capable of enjoying sex is naïve and, in fact, ridiculous. The route to physical and emotional sexual happiness depends on several attainable considerations: reassurance from an understanding partner, willingness to give and accept love, realistically adapting to physical, and ` ageing challenges, and bringing communication to our relationship.

It is said that "sex is the most powerful affirmation in the face of death." Gratifying sex is a process of tenderness and love. With courage, curiosity, and communication, we can experience emotional and physical enjoyment of our and our partner's sexuality and share intimacy until the sun sets. Now, over 60, our sex lives do not belong in the history book of life but, can assume a new vitality when successfully redefined. Sexuality represents life refusing to give in to death.

Chapter 10
Loss and Mood Changes Over 60

Losing close friends affects mood. Parents decline and die creating a vacuum, emptiness, and a wake-up call of a man over 60s' mortality. Boomers are the next generation on deck. With a spouse's death an ill-prepared man must redefine himself now socialising without a partner and dealing with aloneness but, not necessarily loneliness. Classmates and friends are dying. A man's earlier years may feel wistfully gone. Men cannot avoid realising their years are limited. Common mood changes develop over loss, physical, or emotional changes. The right drugs prescribed by a savvy psychiatrist trained in elder psychiatry, can reverse emotional events associated with ageing that are treatable.

> "Getting older is a struggle. I always feel that just under the surface of acceptance and enjoyment of the ageing process is a terrible hysteria just waiting to burst out."
>
>   – Michael Sheen, Actor

This chapter runs the gamut from losing close friends, wives, depression, or a multitude of vicissitudes that may affect our mood. Testosterone is one of the male hormones that may protect us from depression. Over sixty, as testosterone wanes, we are more susceptible to depression. The lifetime prevalence for depression among women ranges from 9 to 26% and for men 5 to 12%. Women report depression more than men. Men and women have an equal prevalence of bipolar disorder. Men have more bipolar 1, the more serious form, associated with hospitalisation and, all too often, psychosis.

Men have higher rates of criminal behaviour, alcoholism, and other addictions. Mental illness and chemical dependence (MICD) co-occur in both sexes. We are just the "bad boys". Completed Suicide is greater in elderly white males than in women, or as the saying goes, "Women try, men do." Men have greater access to guns. Women use pills and their attempt can be a cry for help. Another explanation is that women are more likely to feel depression and ask for help.

In an article, *Men and Depression,* which I wrote with, Dr Paula Clayton, then professor and chair of the Department of Psychiatry at the University of Minnesota School of Medicine, we reported that the death rate by suicide for men was 19.1 per 100,000 compared with 4.9 per 100,000 among women. Suicide can be fast, effective, and lethal for a man – especially for a man who is intoxicated, with less impulse control, and who owns a hunting rifle or handgun.

Suicide is the most painful act for loved ones left behind, blaming themselves and asking, "How could I have prevented his suicide?"

In the dreary early fall or late winter, men and women can experience seasonal affective disorder (SAD), a type of depression related to too little sun. Fortunately, SAD responds to light therapy (10,000 lux, 30–45 minutes a day), psychotherapy, and vitamin D. Antidepressants, especially the selective serotonin inhibitors(SSRIs) can be helpful. At our age, the loss of a loved one can precipitate grief, loneliness, and emptiness that can compound our struggle with ageing and death.

Creative men are at an increased risk for depression. One study showed that 80% of creative writing students at the Iowa Writer's Workshop suffered at least one episode of depression or mania in their lifetime. PBS launched a TV series, *Moods, and Music,* highlighting the link between creativity and mood disorders.

Hitting the mark on a diagnosis of dysphoria in men over sixty is never easy. Depression in older men can masquerade as a character or personality disorder, inattention, or suggest alcohol or drug abuse. In the over-sixty set, depression can look like dementia or Alzheimer's disease. Clinicians refer to this process as "pseudodementia". An underlying emotional issue related to a disturbing work or personal relationship problem may underly depression. Recurring lifelong unipolar depression or bipolar disorder can be at the root of unexplained failures that began in childhood or adolescence, and reoccurring in later life.

A man over 60 with unipolar depression may repeatedly over weeks or months-awaken early, so-called "terminal insomnia". Classically, chronic inability to fall to sleep is a symptom more of an anxiety disorder. Someone, of any age or sex who is depressed may report feeling sad, lacking interest and energy, a weight change, or a sleep disturbance. Someone with depression may also have feelings of unworthiness, hopelessness, self-condemnation, concentration lapses, suicidal ideation, anger, irritability, and hypercritical behaviour.

Midlife is not the only volatile period of a man's life. My earlier book, *Dr D's Handbook: A Guide to Health, Fitness, Living, and Loving, in the Prime of Life* (Wiley & Sons, 1999) speaks to the emotional effects of waning midlife hormones, concomitant alcohol abuse, weight gain or loss, feelings of worthlessness, guilt, poor concentration, or disabling thoughts of death or suicide Men who are depressed have more somatic symptoms such as fatigue, constipation, weight change, or disturbed appetite than women. We may demonstrate psychological symptoms of hopelessness.

A depressed man's moods may cycle during the day, week, month, or year, sometimes reappearing mysteriously later in life. A man who is depressed may have disabling symptoms from agitated depression. We may feel safer expressing our anger at family members we love than at work or play. We may hide from depression with self-directed anger by displacing our anger toward our wife, children, or friends. We are less likely to do so in the workplace. What better distraction from the internal turmoil that is the demon of depression than by fighting with those whom we love, not fearing reprisal as we would from co-workers or a superior.

Secondary depression from an untimely loss is less associated with suicide than endogenous, internal depression, the latter, the genetic variety. It is easy to understand how developing Alzheimer's, Parkinson's, renal, coronary disease, or newly diagnosed cancer, can precipitate depression. Withdrawing from alcohol, drugs, or smoking can produce depression, but is more likely to be short lived and usually lasting only two weeks.

Experiencing an older man in our life's behaviour with such forms of maladaptive often hurtful and uncharacteristic dysfunctional symptoms and behaviours, typical of chronic depression in an older man we love or ourselves – that's hanging on too long-may require some detective work to discover the underlying cause for the problem. There is no fault in calling your on-call clinic nurse or even the crisis line for depression you may be experiencing lasting one or more weeks.

The clinical term, dysthymia – like drug dependency, is an equal opportunity destroyer. That is why, unlike my friend who refuses treatment, most of those with depression can be effectively treated with appropriate antidepressant medications. Acute episodes affecting those with characterological depression, as well as an older man with primary(endogenous) or secondary(exogenous) depression that may have been simmering for over a month, can and should be effectively treated. Unfortunately, often those with characterological difficulties or those men or women who mistakenly believe their depression will dissipate, in many instances, avoid treatment.

Professor Clayton explained that insight-oriented psychotherapy has no positive effect on depression. She opines that it is most often necessary to treat a man with moderate to severe depression; that is, major depressive disorder (MDD), with medication. Others advocate cognitive behavioural therapy (CBT), employing both verbal and behavioural techniques to help patients recognise that negative ideas about themselves are inaccurate. "CBT, given the right circumstances, works," She explains.

Dr Clayton notes the efficacy of interpersonal psychotherapy for managing depressed patients with grief and loss, interpersonal ongoing struggles, or marital disharmony. The feelgood endorphins we all have that – with moderate and consistent exercise, sex, good food, and happy times-usually effectively improve transient depressive symptoms.

Early tricyclic antidepressants that include amitriptyline, nortriptyline, imipramine; desipramine; and doxepin had their place in treating depression. Their annoying side effects include over-sedation, urinary retention, constipation, dry mouth, lowered blood pressure, and arrhythmias. They are rarely used today.

The current treatment of choice for moderate depression is the selective serotonin reuptake inhibitors (SSRIs). Prozac (fluoxetine) got it all started as a sure-fire and less problematic way to treat major depressive disorder (MDD). Then came Celelexa (citalopram), Lexapro (escitalopram), Paxil (paroxetine), and Zoloft (sertraline), and others. On the downside, side effects from the SSRIs include nausea, weight loss, dysfunctional orgasm, or other forms of ED.

Like any mood stabiliser, there are side effects. The good news is that SSRIs, if taken as an overdose, are much less likely to be lethal. Side effects like sexual dysfunction can be a reason older guys decide not to take this class of drugs. Another hidden danger of all the antidepressants is, after initiating a course of therapy for MDD, a patient may just have enough energy to take that final and fatal step, suicide.

Another class of antidepressant are the selective serotonin and norepinephrine reuptake inhibitors (SNRIs). These include Effexor (venlafaxine), Pristiq (desvenlafaxine), and Cymbalta (duloxetine). They, too, are designed to effectively treat depression.

In the event of unmitigated depression lasting over 12 weeks during which a psychiatrist has tried two or three medications that proved unsuccessful, a course of electroconvulsive therapy (ECT) may work. At the present level of technology, it is dependable, safe, and with the least number of side effects. There is only transient memory loss. An estimated 30,000 to 50,000 Americans undergo ECT yearly.

Depression occurs at all stages of a man's life. It affects all rungs of society. It may be a primary condition, or secondary to medical or situational stressors in a man's life. Men over 60 are no exception. Depression, a treatable mood disorder in men over 60, is a potentially dangerous mental health issue that must be recognised and effectively treated.

It is important to discern the difference between primary depression – an inherited dysphoria, from secondary depression, precipitated by a cataclysmic breakup or a life-transforming medical illness. Characterological depression is more of personality disorder, which is an emotionally "built-in" variety.

I would characterise one friend's personality as mercurial with anger, simmering just below the surface, waiting to grab anyone in the way, sometimes myself. Someone with characterological depression, given the right circumstances, is a set-up for suicide. Such an unfortunate turn of events is what may have happened to a dear friend, previously a brilliant private school headmaster. His career had suddenly shifted when he left his delightfully full role in the school, had a brief sojourn with a non-profit health and wellness facility, and assumed an exciting headmaster's position at the American School in Cairo.

Dan had always been quiet and rarely expressed emotions but, appeared to enjoy a life of academic achievement, family harmony, and a love for endurance sports including coaching and cross-country ski racing for many years. It was not unusual for Dan to bike twenty miles to and from school every day. His last note to me described what was happening at his new challenge in Egypt. He described some difficulties that he described as unsolvable. Then there was the news that Dan was dead. His death was sadly reported as a suicide. He had hung himself.

The cues for unmanageable depression were not there. I thought of our times joyfully gathering and boiling down maple syrup on his property. I had memories of laughing as we passed each other on a mountain bike journey in northern Minnesota. Visits with him at his headmaster's office were always rewarding. But I had sensed a sadness and loneliness in Dan. As with many suicides, I was surprised, saddened, and wished I had been in Cairo to support him, as he may have sunk deeper into an underlying depression that was triggered by his new and unsolvable setbacks.

My recent memoir, *Up from the Ashes: One Doc's Struggle with Drugs and Mental Illness* (2018) describes the experiences of a man well over sixty, struggling with another pattern of dysphoria, bipolar disorder. Bipolar disorder is a life of ups and downs in which moods swing between depression and, in the case of bipolar 1, mania with the potential for psychosis often requiring hospital admission. Bipolar 2 has similar dips of depression but lower episodes of mania that are described as hypomania. With different intervals, this disorder can begin in early childhood and, with stressors reaching a kindling point, can ignite in men over sixty. Some mental health problems are hereditary. This is especially true for bipolar disorder and other mental illnesses like schizophrenia.

Bipolar disorder either as bipolar 1 with mania cycling with depression, or bipolar 2 with hypomania the less dangerous form of mania, and a similar level of depression, responds well to lithium. Studies confirm that bipolar disorder can begin in childhood, often confused with hyperactivity, resurface in midlife as solitary depressive episodes, and also can surface in men over 60. Lithium, the original drug for bipolar disorder, can decrease relapses of depression with lower rates of suicides. Thyroid and renal functions in someone taking lithium should be monitored with periodic blood tests.

Both disorders can now be successfully treated especially with antiseizure medications like Neurontin (gabapentin), Depakote (valproic acid), Tegretol (carbamazepine) Trileptal (oxcarbazepine), or Lamictal (lamotrigine). Rarely, is one medication sufficient so psychiatrists add other medications such as an atypical antipsychotic, Seroquel (quetiapine), or Zyprexa (olanzapine) especially for difficulty with sleep.

A more benign variant, cyclothymia, is characterised by racing thoughts, distractibility, and depression. Cyclothymia has smaller spikes and dips and fluctuates yet, can be discomforting and escalate with time. Therapy such as cognitive behavioural therapy (CBT) is reported as helpful. Mood stabilisers such as lithium, antiseizure medications, anticonvulsants like divalproex, oxcarbazepine, and lamotrigine, can help simmer things down.

Atypical antipsychotics such as olanzapine, quetiapine, and risperidone may work if a patent is resistant to the other medications. The SSRI's alone can trigger mania. With time, cyclothymia can morph into either bipolar 1 or 2 disorders. This brief overview should enable us to better detect, intervene, and effectively treat the treatable.

My eighty-year-old friend, "Doc" tells me mental illness runs in his family. Knowing him for half a century, I would suggest that it gallops in his. Faced with his painful lashing out, I have encouraged him countless times to get help and, if recommended, take medications that could stabilise his mercurial mood shifts. He demurs saying that a good cup of coffee, or the sun breaking out of the clouds makes him feel better.

As his friend, I have often been the recipient of his angry mood shifts when he appears depressed, agitated, and lashes out at me. His long-standing and tolerant partner denies there is a problem. She, like families of alcoholics, often are co-dependent. They fail to recognise the eponymous elephant in the living room. Caught up in the dysfunction itself, love ones often blame themselves and believe what is going on is their problem. Doc just shuts down as a way of keeping their relationship together Her denial is, "It works for us," she explains stoically.

My friend may well have a characterological depression; that is, someone who has an underlying depressive personality like my dear and deceased friend, Dan. New outside stressors or emotional setbacks can light an ambient compensated depressive personality beyond the kindling point as it appears to do especially with my friend, "Doc". My struggles with my challenging friend confirm the adage, if you have friends like him, you do not need an enemy. However, I care for him enough that I continue to value his friendship however it might be.

He is eighty-one now and noticeably more fragile. He confesses to me while he was supervising work I was doing on his home. "It's getting tough even for me to sign my name." Just by observing his halting walk or difficulty rising from a chair, I sense he has early Parkinson's. Many of us close to his age deny our mortality or, in Doc's case, struggle not-so-quietly, while denying their worsening disability. He does so by delaying writing his will. Writing one is always something he will do… later.

He has always refused to seek help. Not long ago, his VA doctor ran a parathyroid scan to explain his repeated episodes of kidney stones throughout his adult life. "Bones, moans, and groans" is how doctors describe it. Doctors discovered he had an overactive parathyroid gland due to little tumours on the gland. His hyperparathyroidism in addition to kidney stones and dissolving bone, is associated with emotional issues like "Doc's". After surgery, a parathyroidectomy, his lab tests are normal now. His medical problem exacerbated his underlying characterological depressive personality. In hindsight, his diagnosis is one of exclusion. Has his mood or behaviour changed? Tough call. Probably, not.

Recently and with great emotional difficulty, he sold a town home he was renting out. Then he bought a tumbled-down vintage 50s house on some acreage. "It reminds me of the house I grew up in. I call it 'The Farm'." Selling farm acreage where he has hunted for half a century that is tilled by some local farmers, was another difficult process. My friend has had a full personal and professional life. But now, his age is catching up to him. Much to my surprise, he appears of late to be handling the changes in his life better. The good news and despite physical limitations, he is happy. He has never threatened to kill himself… or, worse yet, me.

Manly, my beloved 91-year-old attorney and dear friend, pushes on with his life despite his wife's passing almost a decade ago. In his words, "It was on a blind date in the summer of 1963 that I met the girl of my dreams. We had thirty years of a beautiful life together. I was not prepared in 1995 when Jan succumbed to metastatic breast cancer. I did not want to believe it – not my heathy, indestructible sweetheart. I was determined to try to be with her throughout the whole process including two surgeries, a bone marrow transplant, visiting countless doctors, and treatment programs making sure that I would always be there for her. She was a strong, determined mother, social worker, and wonderful wife."

As a man in his late sixties, Manly never anticipated Jan's illness would put his love and dedication to the test. "During the 11-years of her illness, her mental strength and wisdom helped me get through what was often a painful ordeal."

Manly has always been an indomitable lawyer, a compassionate father of two adult daughters, and always there for his beloved grandchildren. "I've got to finish all the business I still have before I retire." He continues to enjoy the getaway in Miami he had shared with his wife. "I'm on the condominium board there and in Minneapolis. "I want to retire," he tells me year after year. He always stretches out the deadline when he will retire.

Finally, he closed his office but quickly became of counsel in another. I knew Manly enough to disbelieve him when he said, "I can't wait to get out of here." Come January, he heads for Miami where he also enjoys his life. But he is back for a week in February. Again, I hear, "I've got to finish business." Manly loves life. He appears to savour the pleasure of aloneness or, at least, does not complain about it. He does not impose on his children and, when in town, relishes spending a few weekend days with his two adolescent grandchildren.

He denies feeling lonely. Losing Jan was not easy for Manly. After several abortive attempts at dating, he tells me, "There is no replacement for Jan." To meet for dinner, I still need to alert him a week in advance. "I'm so damned busy," he tells me. My bimonthly dinners before he retired were about discussing life, law, and politics. Over good food, we shared our views of the world. Now, with COVID-19, we meet weekly at an outdoor café. Keep at it, Manly. Alone, yes, but he is never lonely. People should remain positive and emphasise the good things in life despite often-unexpected, sometimes sad circumstances.

According to the National Institute on Alcohol Abuse and Alcoholism (NIAA), alcohol and drug abuse affects up to 17% of those over sixty. Among the baby boomers, addiction issues are expected to reach 5.7 million by 2020. Alcohol is at the front of the pack for addiction. Diagnosing addiction and abuse in older men and women can be difficult. A problem like addiction can mimic behavioural symptoms of depression or medical problems such as diabetes, or endocrine disorders like hyperparathyroidism, as in Doc's case. There are two variants of addiction. One is called the "hardy survivor", the man who has been using and abusing throughout much of his life. The other, "late onset", is someone who becomes addicted or alcoholic de novo in a later part of life.

We must look for triggers such as retirement, passing of a loved one, unexpected poverty, or relocation such as entering a nursing facility. Friends and loved ones need to be aware of alcohol or drug abuse – especially from prescribed ones from doctors for a problem such as insomnia, or self-prescribing in the face of declining physical or emotional health.

An older man, especially into his seventies and eighties, does not metabolise or tolerate alcohol and drugs as when he was younger. Hopefully, he can fall into the hands of a gerontologist who knows the addictive potential and correct dosages of drugs like the frequently addictive benzodiazepines. Not uncommonly, as among younger men, the addict or alcoholic minimises, even lies about their use. Mental illness and chemical abuse (MICD) run hand-in-hand.

The clinician must look for an inciting event that can help explain vague physical symptoms of tiredness, memory loss, or depression in a man over sixty. Faced with observing in an older man memory fluctuations, disturbed sleep patterns; unexplained bruises, possibly from falls or fights; altered eating habits; bad hygiene; or isolating from family or friends, an observant physician or loved ones should address the possibility of addiction or alcoholism.

Specialised treatment programs are available for the older alcoholic or addict. Marc E. Agronin in *How We Age: A Doctor's Journey into The Heart of Growing Old.* has one vignette after another how, as a geriatric psychiatrist, he makes one after another successful diagnosis that improves the life of his patients. His perspective is one of understanding correctable issues relating to complex memory or behavioural changes.

Sir William Osler, the consummate clinician, who helped found Johns Hopkins Hospital in the early twentieth Century, advised, "The good physician treats the disease, the great physician treats the patient who has the disease." The National Institute of Alcohol Abuse and Alcoholism (NIAA) advises that adults over 65 be limited to one standard drink (12 ounces of beer, 4-5 ounces of wine, or one-and- a half ounces of distilled spirits per day or seven standard drinks per week, and no more than three drinks on special occasions. I advise zero tolerance: NO driving for a man over 60 after any alcohol. I have conflicting feelings about pigeonholing treatment centres that treat older individuals separately. I believe that issues of transference between younger and older patients can be productive rather than interfering with either party's treatment success. Elders and younger men and women bring their special gifts and perspectives to treatment. 18% of treatment centres feel that the ageing population benefits from a segregated recovery setting and are specifically designed for older adults. The late New York Times columnist, James Carr, described addiction as a demon chronically simmering and lurking in the basement doing push-ups and ready to jump.

Drug abusing among the elderly ranges from abusing either intentionally or unintentionally prescribed medications. Among individuals fifty-seven to eighty-five, 37.1% of men take over five prescription medications. Benzodiazepines are the most prescribed psychiatric medication among all adults – rates prescribed are 15.2 to 32.0% for older adults. Drug interactions must be considered with every prescription. Confusion taking medications is always a hazard. Most older men or women can benefit from a pill organiser. I am beginning to realize that means me.

If in doubt, refer to the DSM criteria for substance use disorder (SUD). Screening for substance abuse of any kind should be an integral part of all physician exams and; especially, yearly physicals. The most common screening tool for substance misuse is the CAGE. The study that has the most thorough exploration of substance abuse in older men was published by Alexis Kuerbis et al in *Clin Geriatr Med*. 2014 Aug; 30(3):629–654, an exhaustive metanalysis.

So be it. Emotional challenges and addiction are no stranger to men over 60. Regardless, all the problems described in this chapter have answers and solutions. Be aware. Don't fear. Rather, ask a loved one or your physician if any of the signs and symptoms I have described representing inner or outside turmoil, confusion, insomnia, or sexual disappointments that are boiling inside you become black beasts Remember, being over 60 may bring on painful crises but, if resolved, can insure that passing the 60 mark will provide a fruitful episode in your life.

Chapter 11
Stretching

Meditative stretching before, during, and after aerobic and strength workouts helps avoid injuries, hastens recovery, and relieves stress. Make it a must for your training program. Some say they even sleep better after stretching. Strengthening lengthens tiny muscle fibrils up to 150%. Young athletes rupture muscle. Men over 60 rip tendons and ligaments. Stretching can help avoid ripping an Achilles, biceps, or hamstring while enhancing flexibility and improving blood supply and oxygenation to injured muscles. The text provides a medley of solo and partnered stretches. Don't forget facial muscles. After stretching, a massage therapist can carefully further improve now more pliable muscles.

My poodle stretched every morning, why shouldn't I?

"I never struggled with injury problems because of my preparation – in particular, my stretching."
—   Edwin Moses two-time Olympic Gold in the 400 Meter with a World Record four times

Just because you are over 60 does not mean you can't still push your body. Studies support that exercise – aerobic or anaerobic – can make our mature years more enjoyable. Begin your exercise session with stretching.

Dr D's Handbook: *A Guide to Health, Fitness, Living, and Loving in the Prime of Life*, explains how a good exercise program that includes stretching will enhance the quality of a man's life after 40. As we cruise past 60, it is vital now as ever to continue a complete exercise program that includes stretching. Combined with aerobic and resistance training stretching will make exercise more enjoyable, safer, and enhance recovery.

Stretching before, during your warm-up, and during your cool down prevents injury. Stretch, stretch, stretch.

Stretching works at the microscopic level, lengthening tiny muscle fibrils. Collectively, power lies in the large muscle groups. Collectively, power lies in larger muscle groups. Experts describe properties of muscle when it reacts to a stimulus; with contraction, muscles shorten and thicken. The good news is that muscles can stretch 150% and rebound.

Among the older set, tendons, ligaments, and connective tissue are not as elastic as muscle and more easily injured. The opposite is true for younger athletes who rip muscles. Tendons and ligaments do not stretch. Instead, they snap and rupture like uncooked spaghetti. We must carefully stretch connecting muscles that are attached to tendons, ligaments, and connective tissue. For the older athlete stretching helps us avoid injury, pain, and the inability to keep at it.

Imagine a grandfather taking off after his grandson. He suddenly feels like a bullet has hit him in the back of his heel. He may well have ripped an Achilles tendon where it inserts into the heel at the calcaneus bone. Pushing against a wall or telephone pole stretching his calves might have avoided this injury. Note, that there are two calf muscles, the inner soleus, and the larger outer gastrocnemius, that need individual stretching, accomplished by lowly sliding back the ball of the stretching foot behind you from an almost vertical placement into 45 degrees toe to ground as the calf is being stretched-first the inner then the hefty outer muscle, as the ball of your foot moves backward.

Protecting the joints and ligaments is all about stretching so muscles do not hyperextend or over flex. Putting extreme torque on vulnerable ligaments or tendons like the Achilles, the hamstring, a biceps, can be a prescription for ending your sport season. Gentle extension by slow stretching can prevent injuring more vulnerable and hard-to-heal tendons, classically, calf, hamstring or biceps muscle tendons.

Think Out of the Box

Painless slow stretching should be your goal. This is the time for low weights and avoiding pain. Avoid activating an injured muscle too soon. Take plenty of down time to convalesce an injured muscle. Forget the "No Pain no gain" myth. Do some slow stretches to enhance the blood supply and oxygenation to injured muscles. Gradually, you can add light weights as you increase resistance and up repetitions.

Are you ready to go? Please do not quit yet. You have gotten this far in the book. Regular exercise can help us grow older younger. Consistent exercise makes me happy: those endorphins again However, I must take care to consistently stretch. Often, if I am feeling pain in my calf, my groin, low back, or hamstring-even as my exercise has already begun-I will stop and do another stretch. We, as older athletes, for all the reasons given above, cannot do too much stretching.

For starters, grab your gym bag, bring your water bottle, and wait until after you exercise to eat your big meal. Something light before exercise is fine – a banana, an apple, a stick of string cheese. Eating a big meal can divert vital blood your heart needs to pump vital oxygen and glucose to your body and brain. Go light at first.

Plan to stretch before and after exercise. This has never been my strong suit, but do as I say not as I might not-so religiously do. Testimony why plenty of want-a-be athletes end up bailing from an exercise program is due to a gonzo start and then getting a pulled hamstring, a painful torn rotator cuff, or an overstretched inguinal ligament. I have learned how helpful stretching can be before, after, or even, while exercising especially once I have warmed up. Old habits are hard to break, and that includes forgetting to stretch, which then can compromise the flexibility needed to avoid injury. Stretching prepares ligaments, tendons, and muscles and protects against the torque often experienced in vigorous exercise.

Stretching – especially post-exercise, decreases recovery time and muscle discomfort that might prevent any athlete, new or more fit, from continuing exercising. Bob Anderson, author of *Stretching*, points out that most people spend too much time exercising and too little time stretching. Anderson, applying yoga that has been around since well before Western medicine, preaches his mantra to athletes of every discipline. "Stretch!"

I remember well running with Bob up the sizeable hill behind his lovely, secluded home near Colorado Springs, where I was volunteering at The United States Olympic and Paralympic Training Center. The run must have been tough because I remember blowing out the back of my running shoes. But, afterward – under Bob's discerning eye, we damn well stretched.

An athlete ought quickly learn which muscles are hurting, what muscles to use, and which ones need a break. Stretching allows anyone – neophyte, or high-powered athlete – to stay in the game, resume exercising sooner, and maintain consistent painless performance. Such a simple meditative technique makes exercising more fun, safer, and yes, a nurturing stress reliever. You may just sleep better!

General Stretching Rules

First, do a short run, a half-hour on the elliptical, a swim, or your call and, voila, muscles, now warmed up, become more pliable and elastic.

- **Avoid rapid or jerky** movements. Do not bounce!
- **Stretch to** a significant end resistance **but,** NOT painful. Hold it for 20 to 30 seconds.
- **Go slow** – this is a perfect opportunity to get mellow.
- **Stretch opposing muscles** – like your hamstrings versus your quads.
- **Breathe** - The Ayuvedic principle, "In from the nose, out from the mouth", applies just as in yoga, and is helpful once you begin lifting or running.
- **Stretch regularly,** whether exercising or not. Try three times a week for starters.

Types of Stretching
Begin with an easy stretch of your groin muscles
The Achilles Stretch

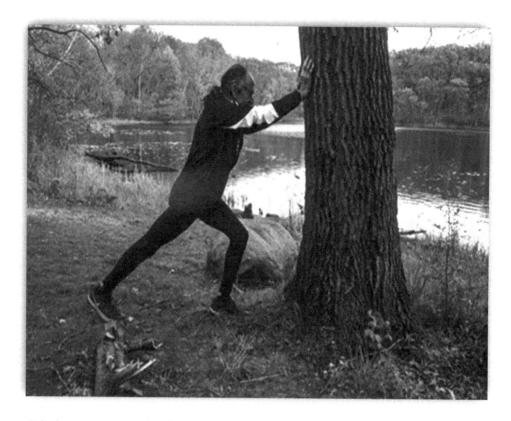

It is the strongest tendon in the body and allows people to push off while walking, running and jumping. People talk about ripping one or both Achilles tendons that feels like someone shot them right above the heel. Unexpected rips and a rupture of this calf tendon can occur after a quick, stop-and-start activity such as a sudden run on the racket or tennis court for a low ball at the net, an unexpected step off the curb, or after a quick sprint after your grandson.

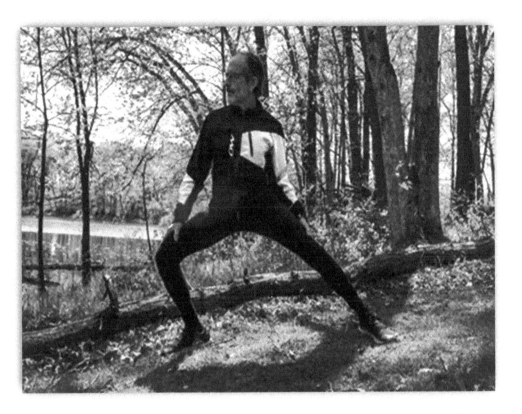

Incidentally, the word on the street is that taking care of a toddler is as hard a physical challenge as being a NFL tight end.

- Sit with your legs in front of you flat on the floor. Gently grasp your toes pulling them comfortably toward your body. Hold 20 seconds then slowly release.
- Alternatively, stand as if you're trying to push the building, tree, or telephone pole down with your arms extended hard against the building

6–12 inches above shoulder level and your legs behind you, the closest foot flat and up on your toes of your back foot. As you stretch you can move your back foot farther to move the stretch down your calf and into your Achilles tendon. Switch legs. **Go slow.**

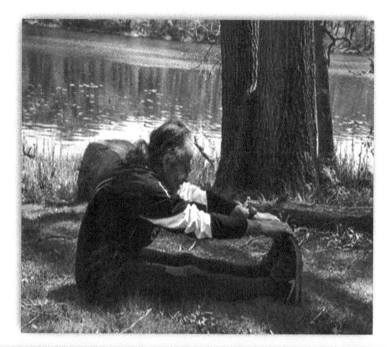

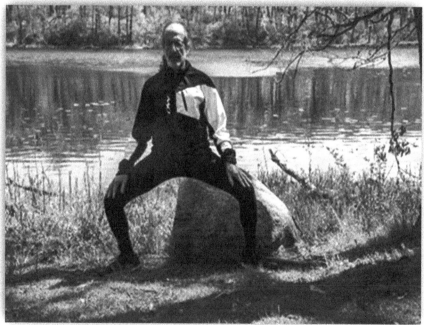

Quadriceps and Groin Stretches

Lying back with your legs apart, gently twist and pull back and toward either side feeling the comfortable pull at your inguinal ligament

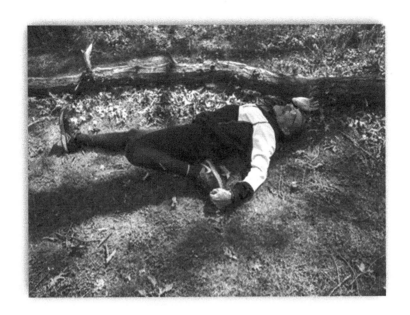

Quadriceps and Groin Stretches

Sitting or lying, gently drop your knees to either side. Another nice way to stretch your hamstrings and groin muscles. Lie on your back with your legs straight then crossing your feet and bending your knee. Gently cross the bent knee over your

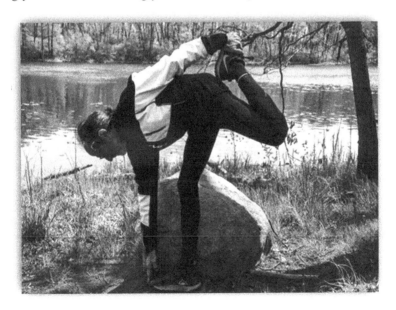

thigh so you can feel the stretch on your rotator and hamstring insertions.

The Pelican Stretch

Stand next to a wall or pole that you can use for balance. Slowly bend forward with your body resting against the wall if necessary while reaching as far as you can with your fingers to the floor in front of your left ankle stretching your hamstring as you pull backward holding your right ankle by your right glut stretching your opposite quad. Two birds (muscles) with one stone

A Lone or Partnered Hamstring Stretch

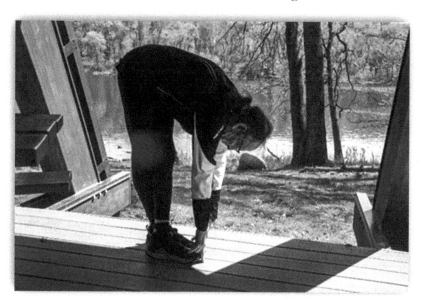

Sitting back-to-back grabbing your partners flexed arms from behind, take turns carefully flexing your upper bodies forward and back. Great again for a guided quadriceps, hamstring, and groin stretch. (Not pictured)

- Standing, cross one leg in front of the other, then carefully, bend forward, feeling the stretch of your hamstring muscle and insertion. Repeat with the other leg. Sit flat as you can, your back at 90 degrees with the ground with your legs about 45 degrees apart and slowly reach as far forward as you can to hold your ankle as you lean forward to stretch your hamstring muscle and its insertions. With all hamstring stretches, do not bounce. Increase your stretch slowly
- Standing, cross one leg in front of the other, then carefully, bend forward, feeling the stretch of your hamstring muscle and insertion. Repeat with the other leg. Sit flat as you can, your back at 90 degrees with the ground with your legs about 45 degrees apart and slowly reach as far forward as you can to hold your ankle as you lean forward to stretch your hamstring muscle and its insertions. With all hamstring stretches, do not bounce. Increase your stretch slowly.

Hip Rotator Stretches

With two persons your feet touching, both of your legs 45 degrees apart with your hands clasped, gradually push each other's legs apart. This is one stretch when it is important your partner's a friend(Not pictured)

- Sit. Grab an ankle, and gently pull it back and alongside your buttock, slowly lowering your upper body backward. Great for stretching the quadriceps. Go slow and only if comfortable.

Lower Back Stretches

- The key to maintaining back comfort and avoiding injury is by strengthening core. More about that later in the strength chapter.
- Remember to concentrate on your posture. That is the best way to avoid "senile posture" defined as the gradual pitching forward of your head. Who knows, maybe, keeping an eye on the upcoming terrain ahead may be why you bend forward as an unconscious protective effort to avoid falling. But, better to avoid a fall than that your posture gets style points.

Stand tall, your hands stretching toward the sky. Carefully, with your palms forward, lean as far back as possible then dropping your arms toward the front. Go slow.

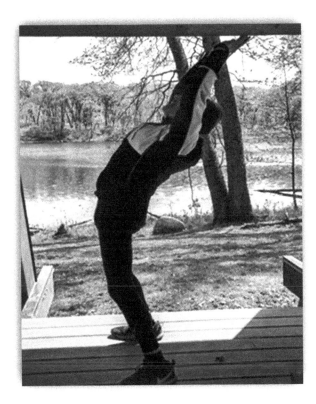

"The Lion" in yoga is an effective technique in which you get down on all fours. Drop your back, slowly thrusting your abdomen toward the floor breathing out, looking as far up and toward the sky searching for the sun. It is surprisingly fun to stick your tongue out. Then, in a few seconds, arch your back, breathing in as you drop your head stretching your neck muscles.

- Lie flat on your back. Grab your ankles from outside your knees, pulling your heels to the base of your buttocks. Now, and, with great care, roll back-and-forth front-to-back allowing all your vertebrae to get a private little massage during each part of the roll but take care not to overdo the roll to include your neck.

Your biceps are especially vulnerable. Muscles shorten, ligaments and tendons weaken and lose power with age. A "Popeye" muscle can occur suddenly from a rip at the lower biceps tendon-leaving a severed ball instead of a normal

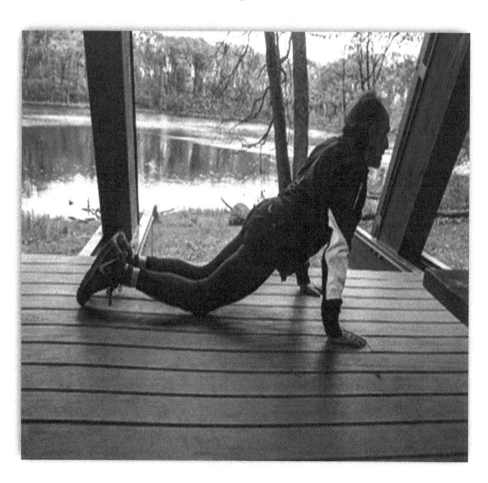

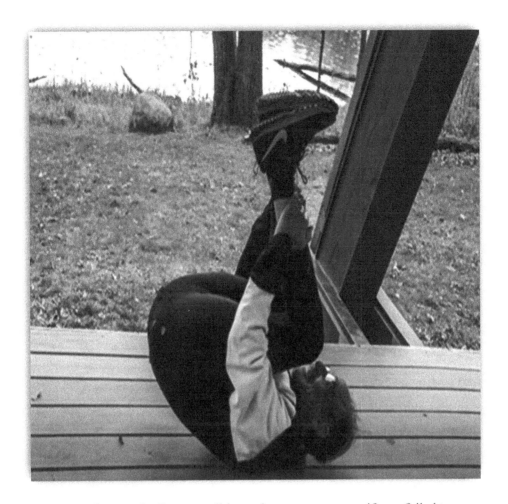

biceps. Such a surgically correctible tendon tear can occur if you failed to sufficiently stretch and ripped off the lower biceps insertion injuring an otherwise powerful muscle.

Using a soft bungee to flex and extend your biceps and triceps can prevent the painful pop of ripping the distal tendon of the biceps as it inserts into the radial head at your elbow.

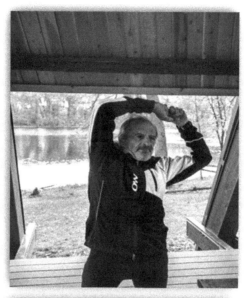

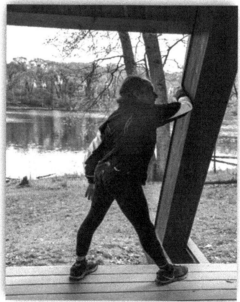

Pectoral Muscle Stretches

The pectoral muscle stretch are the arms horizontally at a 45 degree angle from the floor as you extend the stretch of your arms feeling the front pectoral chest muscles loosening. Need that picture here.

Stand or sit with your arms horizontal to the floor outstretched straight at 90 degrees from your body and pull your arms back so you can feel these wide chest muscles stretch. Then, with your Pecs muscles warmed up and stretched, it's time to do those push-ups and pull-ups.

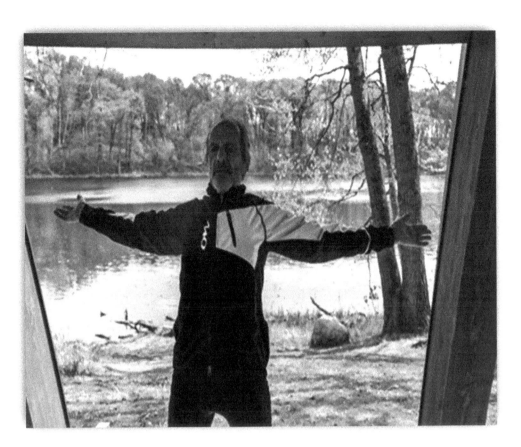

Trapezius (Your "Traps"), Cervical spine, and Paraspinal neck Muscles

- This is the wide muscle running down the back of your neck onto your shoulders. Rotating your neck around with each individual stretch and relaxing your cervical vertebrae and muscles. Think like an owl as you place the palm of your hand against your chin, the back and sides of your chin, respectively. applying resistance to all four side of your head.

- Opposing muscles on the opposite side of the neck which can save you from a bad sports whiplash

- Pressing the back of your head against the wall lying relaxing and flattening your vertebrae or pushing forward, placing the heel of your hand against your chin, or pushing against the flat of your hand on the side of your head, can stretch both side of the trapezius as well as the tendons holding your spine in place

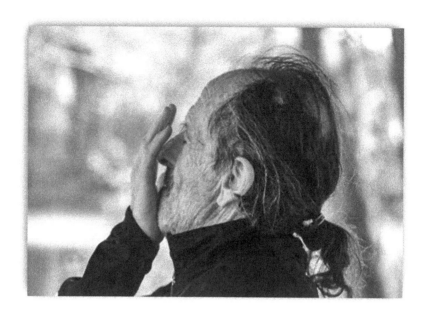

This is a fine way to counter unavoidable arthritic changes which compress cervical vertebrae.

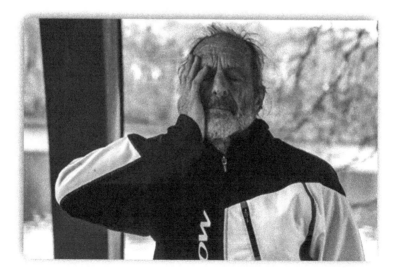

My own cervical vertebrae look like they have been through the Sinai Campaign yet mostly pain free due to these neck flexing techniques against resistance. Stretching by flexing opposing muscles and sliding and flattening the cervical muscles has helped eliminate arthritic pain that epidural cortisone shots did not touch. Thank you, physical therapists who taught me these techniques.

Facial Muscles Stretches

- Just get in front of your bathroom mirror for a before and after. Tense versus relaxed. First, check out the ravages of ageing – for me, years of wind, sleet, and snow cross country skiing – the beauty and the beast of competitive ski racing.
- Now, try 15 seconds contracting all your facial muscles. Keep breathing in through the nose, out from the mouth meanwhile relaxing your face. Stick your tongue out like you're in "kiss." While you are at it, for a moment, you are an Indian guru.

You have discovered a far healthier and surely less addictive stress reliever than alcohol or narcotics but the judicious use of an anti-inflammatory or a minor pain reliever such as an acetaminophen may assist some minor discomfort. I suggest avoiding the former for an acute injury as it may cause more swelling.

Feel free to scream while you are stretching unless you fear the neighbours will call the police. The better the athlete, the more likely he or she is likely to stretch. The most successful ones may practice yoga or stretching exercises as much as an hour daily. Try stretching in the sauna or hot tub, especially after an exercise session. The Russian ski team chose ice baths. Ouch!

Consider incorporating stretching into your massage appointments. Specific stretches such as the ones described above may make you feel better before, during, and, after exercising. The perks are that you will also feel more relaxed performing most other stressful activities.

There are specific exercise movements – I like to call them "range of motion" manoeuvres, that can utilise complimentary muscle groups around challenging joints such as the shoulder and knee. Regarding the knee, patellofemoral exercises strengthen and stretch opposing muscle groups that comprise this hinge joint. The quads are attached to the kneecap from above and extend the lower leg. Calf muscles under and behind the knee do the work flexing the foot. Remember the rips we can experience with too much torque on the Achilles tendon. Hamstrings are equally vulnerable.

The front lower leg muscle, the tibialis anterior, in its surrounding sheath, performs its job extending the foot and benefits from stretching. An exercise prescription, stretching opposing muscles; the quadriceps (stronger) versus hamstrings (weaker); the anterior tibialis (weaker) versus calf muscles (stronger), respond favourably to stretching. With injuries – Range of motion exercises such as patella-femoral ones you can perform just sitting, lying, and standing or rotator cuff manoeuvres using a simple pully, can prevent muscle injuries and avoid more difficult-to-heal tendon and ligament tears around the knee and shoulder, respectively, to which we, as older men are prone.

Another example of a joint we can protect, rehabilitate, and alleviate pain is by stretching as well as strengthening the surrounding muscles around the and rotator cuff. This is another Achilles heel, as it were. The shoulder is a ball in a one-sided socket joint. It is vulnerable – with the wrong fall on an outstretched arm – to dislocation impingement, repeat dislocation, and rotator cuff tears. We, as athletes of any level – even weekend warriors-can strengthen the deltoid, the broad muscle enveloping the shoulder joint, and still-intact rotator cuff muscles with range of motion exercises including a device as simple as a homespun pulley attached to a towel rack or clamped to the top of your bathroom door. If you have not totally ripped too many rotator cuff muscles, an exercise like this can help you avoid the orthopaedist's scalpel and months of immobilisation. A chronically painful shoulder warrants a visit to a sports-minded physician for an exam and potentially shoulder x-rays, and, if indicated, a MRI. Hopefully a referral to physical therapy should the pulley exercises not suffice.

I know, it has worked for me and I'm sure my rotator cuff has had more than one hit. Such an advisement as the overhead motion noted above may seem counter intuitive. Many rehabilitation experts eschew overhead range of motion exercises since an athlete's painful or frozen shoulder more may often results from the repetitive overhead motions in many sports. This technique has worked for me.

You can stretch out a weakened rotator cuff capsule just by using opposing extended arms holding an exceptionally soft bungee or pliable line in both hands that can go around a towel rack and lifting one horizontally straightened arm to ninety degrees over your head as you gently resist the pull with your opposite arm. With one arm up and vertical, the other arm outstretched and ONLY down to a position horizontal or 45 degrees to the ground at shoulder level allows a movement that can amazingly stretch a painful and frozen rotator cuff muscle or tendon This is NOT about weights but rather about range of motion with a stretch backward with each lift. MRI documented subscapularis, supraspinatus, teres minor, or infraspinatus muscles comprising the rotator cuff if with significant full tears may warrant more aggressive orthopaedic evaluation and further care including surgery if indicated.

My advice is that you can carefully work an injured muscle, strained tendon, or inflamed ligament but, depending on severity – stretch gently and begin higher repetitions with light weights, or just stretching with a very flexible bungee cord. Such a prescription increases blood flow to injured muscles. In the acute phase of any muscle or tissue injury, trainers advise resting, icing, compression with an ace wrap, and elevating. I am also advising active but nonpainful movements rather than just quitting. Stretch and stay active.

There is no reason to believe "no pain no gain". Directed stretching promotes heeling, mitigates pain and shortens recovery time. It feels good too! For the acute phase of an injury ice first. After 72 hours, heat or, better yet, contrast therapy – 15 minutes of ice, then 15 minutes of heat – increases blood flow and helps injured muscles heal faster. It is important to cover your heating source with a towel to avoid burning. As you feel more comfortable and do not have pain, gradually increase activity, speed, and resistance. Every aspect of your exercising will improve with stretching. Stretching will increase the blood supply to your muscles which, in turn, can better oxygenate painful injured muscles. Wonderfully, consistent stretching can be a zen-like compliment to aerobic and resistance activities. Stretching also will also get those endorphins flowing!

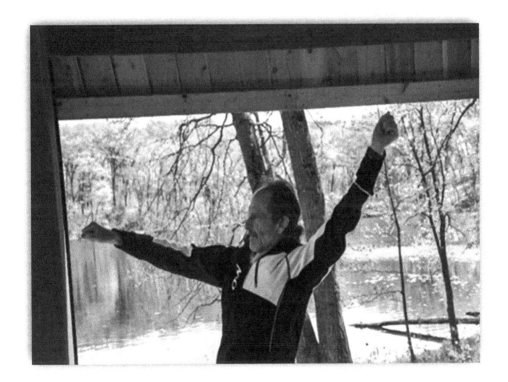

Chapter 12
The Strength Training Mantra

Strength training three times a week slows losing muscle mass, strength, and power. Buy some weights and set up a circuit course on your back deck or hit the gym for machines and free weights. Different methods use isometric, isotonic, and isokinetic techniques. Isometric is the plank. Isotonic lengthens muscle against resistance. Isokinetic on machines, shortens targeted muscles at constant speed and range of motion. Do progressive resistance to fatigue. Start low and slow. After a warmup do a circuit of three sets with ten repeats. You can increase the resistance per set. A strong core makes a strong back.

"Strength does not come from physical capacity – it comes from indomitable will."

– Mahatma Ghandi

Let us start with strength. As we age, especially past 60, or even younger, cardiac performance measured by cardiac output as well as ejection fraction decline. Similarly, muscle mass begins its inevitable decline over the same timeline. As I wrote earlier, we need to delay muscle wasting measured in strength and power.

It is so easy to shove strength training to the side as we jump into DOING whatever sport makes us feel so good. It makes sense, however, to set up a realistic power-enhancing program – not one that could strain or injure muscles – but one that will enhance our chosen sport. Make it fun. I am not averse to utilising work around the house as one available option. You will appear engaged and, take the brownie points when you can.

My friend, Len Sher, who cross country trains hard t also found time to shingle his roof last summer. He is a retired housing inspector but, at 77, was hefting 50-pound boxes of shingles on a ladder up to his roof. I am not an advocate for men our age climbing up on ladders, roofs, or trees. Climbing up and down a ladder or painting inside or outside your house saves money you would pay to the gym. You save money as you enhance your power and strength. Another option is tweaking regular activities like walking or running up and down hills by wearing ankle weights or a weight vest. Ride a tank of a bike rather than one weighing less than a toaster around the local parks. That can make your ride more demanding.

Strong and defined muscles in a man over 60 not only can maintain an enviably sculpted torso – even a twelve pack-but, more importantly, enhance endurance. Your training can be specific or not, but best if consistent. Varying how you exercise makes your fitness choices enjoyable rather than tedious. You can modify your regular year-round strengthening schedule to maintenance during periods of more vigorous days. On your off days try an easy run. Switching from singles to doubles on the tennis, or pickle ball court.

Try swimming some laps. Oh, my, that is work even if you grew up on the Jersey shore as I did, riding the waves. Rest days are important especially after a day of heavy lifting, competition, or a longer work-out. I take it easy on the weekends taking easy walks with Nada, my partner, and, course my now deceased Saidie, the rescue poodle. More is not always better. Everything gets flipped around if you're racing on the weekends. Careful, if you're still working all week lest you fall into the weekend warrior pattern, then spending the next several days for recovery.

After downsizing to a condominium or apartment, you may lose those pick-up strength workouts like shovelling snow or raking leaves. That is a perfect reason to hit the gym on a regular basis or, if you are really disciplined, set up your own program at home on the back deck, or in the basement. A few summers back, I got creative and accrued plenty of fitness exercise painting a friend's barn. What better way to build expendable income while exercising? But do not fall off the ladder. Dragging countless bundles of cut buckthorn can be better than thirty minutes on the elliptical, but the latter can accrue points from your partner. A happy wife or partner makes for a happy life.

Come summer, clearing scrub wood at your cabin, and hauling it to the burn pile is a muscle builder. Unexpected work at someone else's cabin is something else. My friends from college days have renamed my classmate David's cabin "Slave Island". No one gets a free weekend at his New Hampshire getaway. Yet, a soft bed, a tranquil lake, and gourmet cabin-cooked food entices a revolving list of those sufficiently naïve to join his cabin work force expecting a weekend in a hammock. Look at it as an unexpected but enjoyable strength training for my comrades over 75.

Sufficient opportunities for your own strength program are out your back door. Simple resistance exercises can strengthen shoulders, your long back muscles, and develop a strong core of lower and upper "abs". Incline push-ups require only the elevated edge of your deck. If your shoulders can handle it, try them at 35-degrees head down, toes up on the edge of the deck. Installing an expansion bar on the inside casement to your bathroom door is a convenient bar for pull-ups. Voila! Now you have two convenient ways to strengthen your shoulders, arms, core, and upper and lower abdominal muscles.

Keep in mind that strengthening your core is the base of the pyramid for building strength. The abdominal muscles are divided into envelopes of muscles separated by horizontal bands of connective tissues around your muscles that make up a 12 pack. In me it is a two-pack. The upper abdominal muscle respond to crunches that you can do on an incline board with your feet strapped in at the top of the board whereas, the lower abdominal muscles get stronger using the same incline board but then lifting your straightened legs to a 45 degree angle off the lower part of the board. To the horizontal or, if you are really tough to vertical. An easier version of this exercise is to skip an incline and just lie flat on your back then lifting your legs up 35-degrees.

What is muscular strength? It is the amount of force a muscle can exert against any resistance. Strength training is all about POWER. Strengthening neglected muscles not necessarily required in your sport protects those that are crucial. Strength training is not only about primary muscles but also about less used complementary ones. Surprisingly, lower weights with more repetitions can create stronger and, surprisingly, larger muscles like your biceps.

There are two ways to thread the needle. One is to progressively load a muscle, forcing it to work at increasingly greater demand. The alternative is doing lighter work but increase the repetitions. Some muscle groups respond to one or the other better. For instance, legs respond better to overload training; with heavier weights. Abdominals respond best to low resistance, high repetition. However, each technique can replace the other for specific athletic needs.

The overload principle, also called progressive resistance, is to increase the weight as we get stronger. Sage advice is going low and slow and incrementally "stacking weights" – carefully increasing the weight but always avoiding straining too hard, or, worse yet, feeling pain. We best exercise muscle groups at 80% of maximum. We can develop adequate strength with exercise as low as 60% intensity.

Exercising increases muscle definition as well as strength. Unless your goal is to become a body builder, forget it. There is no advantage to bulk that may adversely affect flexibility. This admonition does not hold for prisoners with little else to occupy their time between "the yard" and their cells; and who distract themselves building huge biceps, and triceps – "curls for the girls". Ask your favourite lady if big muscles turn her on. Emotional strength wins all the time.

Just take a glance at a Kenyan or Ethiopian winner of the Boston Marathon. Bulky muscles do not win a distance race. A local running coach surprised me when he was sceptical if strength training makes runners faster. Strength training of an endurance athlete is about higher repetitions and lower weights. An athlete and his trainer must be mindful of the interplay between stressing a muscle to the point of fatigue or, worse yet, an injury. The difference can be a fine line.

Take the "no pain, no gain" concept with a grain of *assault*. I am not particularly impressed with a weightlifter boasting about how much weight he can lift, press, or squat. A measure of success is not necessarily the ability to bench press one's grandmother plus 150 pounds. Let us hope grannie is not overweight because that's when all bets are off. Rather than a he-man build, tell me about the marathoner who placed in the top three in their age group or how well you did in the last charity golf tournament you played?

An effective resistance technique you can follow is the overload principle or of progressively increasing the weight with each set. I like to start with a comfortable weight and, over three sets, reach fatigue when my muscles begin to struggle—but not hurt!. This technique can provide enough specificity to improve your training intensity, your training velocity, and the pattern of your movements. Let us just describe your efforts as an art form of strength and power training.

There are three methods for developing strength.
- Isometric
- Isotonic (concentric, or eccentric)
- Isokinetic

Isometric
Remember the Canadian Air force exercises that we did as prisoners in our dorm rooms in the 1970s? This is an activity done by holding muscles in a fixed position for a length of time while maintaining tension. The Royal Canadian Air Force Exercise Plans, 5BX-Five Basic Exercises-published by Bill Orban in 1961. concluded that, "Long periods of exercise did not necessarily lead to significant improvement." The plan required but 11 minutes and the recipe in book form sold 23 million copies in Canada alone.

This fitness program can be a healthy "quick-fix" that you can take with you down to Santa Fe or Sun City. Another age-old meditative exercise, yoga, employs similar isometric techniques. The Plank is one such position in which you hover on extended arms, palms on the floor, legs apart, straight out behind you, toes to the ground In the privacy your yoga room, you can effectively and effectively strengthen your core. Any barre class integrates The Plank that also can act as a balance and strength act when either opposite leg and arm extends to further toughen abdominal muscles.

Isotonic
This muscle-building technique is either concentric or eccentric contractions against a constant or variable resistance. This is described as a three-step program of five to 10 repetitions three to five days a week, but designed to work muscles to fatigue by the last rep.

- Concentric contraction. The muscle shortens while overcoming a constant resistance.
- Eccentric contraction. The muscles lengthen under a constant resistance. Concentric is generally preferred.

Isokinetic
We are talking about using the machines at the gym. This method allows muscles to develop maximal tension while shortening at a constant speed over a complete range of motion on quiet machines rather than the banging and crashing of the pumping iron set in the free weight room at the back of the gym. Such techniques, under carefully controlled settings, effectively simulates and safely strengthens muscles.

Isotonic

Exercise physiologist, Bob Moffatt, PhD, explains that the principles for building strength and endurance are related to isotonic strength training. Alternately perform three sets of 10 repetitions on machines in the gym or on an elliptical at home every other day from three to five days a week at a comfortable pace, carefully avoiding slapping weights on the machines or yanking muscles in the recovery phase. This approach has comfortably helped me develop greater strength both for everyday physical activities and cross country skiing

I advocate circuit training; including your entire body, one body part after the other, moving from machine to machine in a regular pattern while combining anaerobic lifting with aerobic speed doing three sets and 10 to 20 rep at each station. The goal of this training method of a fast circuit is a great way to develop increased muscular strength while boosting aerobic capacity. Travel through a 6 to 10 station circuit non-stop, and repeat this circuit workout two to three times or more per week. Maximise repetitions at 40–60% of maximal strength, with a 15 to 30 seconds rest between each station. Like interval training, this approach also enhances fast-twitch muscles that are crucial for greater speed.

The whole point of strengthening our bodies is to make them feel better and stronger, allow us to engage in sports more safely with less injury, and, most importantly, have fun while getting stronger. Strengthening opposing muscle groups and, among all parts of our bodies, develop greater strength, can help eliminate and rehabilitate muscle, tendon, and ligament injury. Enhancing complementary muscle groups as, for example, the mighty gastrocnemius (thigh) muscle versus the more touchy and more-frequently injured hamstring muscle, can help you avoid injury that invariably will produce or prolong recovery.

Most Medicare supplemental senior health programs wisely subsidise health club membership. Exercising alone does not always replace a more gregarious option at your nearby health club. In retirement, the a trip to the gym can replace the conviviality of your past work environment. Alternatively, those who exercise alone can substitute exercise machines and gym technology with the accessible resistance exercises on the back deck using our own weight with good old standbys: push-ups, pull-ups, leg or body lifts on an incline board, or just stair climbing at home or work that I previously suggested. Try free weights or elastic bands of variable resistance you can use anywhere.

I strengthen my core, my arms and my legs using my home-built roller board on the back deck (two two-by fours, a sheet of plywood for the deck of the board, with runners to hold in place a sled you can lie, sit, or kneel on with four rollers from the hardware store at all four corners of the sled.). Voila, terrific upper body strengthening. I use mine as well for incline sit-ups and leg lifts that strengthen both tiers of abdominal muscles as described above. A bar on the closet or bathroom casement door can clinch the deal for pull-ups. The goal is making exercise fun, convenient, and effective.

My friend, "Doc Adams", faced with increasing proximal muscle weakness, imbalance, and a shuffling gait, exults how aerobic and resistance exercising has reduced his infirmities – not totally but enough to make his life safer and more

122

vital. What better way to reduce stress and loneliness or just get out of the house and head to the gym? It's like AA. All you may need is some like-minded friends who appreciate staying vigorously alive and sober, in this case fit.

One friend, Toby, has an exercise and coffee work-out group combining exercise and kibitzing. After working out there's always an opportunity to laugh about ageing comparing war (exercise) past injuries at a coffee house. Better to laugh than to cry. Those of us in the medical set liken such a gathering of those over 60 to our clinical pathological conferences (CPCs) – a "guess the disease" medical conferences.

Frederick Hatfield and March Krotee in *Personalized Weight Training for Fitness and Athletics from Theory to Practice* effectively describe the anatomy and physiology of muscle groups. Remember, younger guys pull muscles, whereas older men rip tendons or ligaments that are no longer as pliant as with younger guys.

You should strengthen opposing muscle groups as, for example, thighs ("quads") versus more vulnerable hamstrings as you did when you were stretching. Develop calf strength and flexibility so you will avoid ripping an Achilles tendon at the insertion to the heel. Strengthen your hamstrings, with hamstring curls but, be careful not to overdo the weight or make ballistic movements.

It is all about core and more! Your back thinks so. I advise anyone with constant or repeat back strain-pain-injury to check out their waistline. Remember, guys, we are the apples, the ladies are the pears. More likely, we may have caught a case of "Dunlap's Disease" -when your stomach "dun-lap's" over your belt. It is more than an omen. For the long haul, start with rudimentary crunches. Sit-ups, leg lifts can tighten up your abdomen and help stabilise your back.

For balance as well as strength training try a Bosu ball; first on two feet and later one standing on the platform of the half ball, and for balance keeping a wall or a partner within an arm's length. With a little practice and confidence, always on the ball of your foot, you can begin squats on the flat surface of the Bosu ball. These exercises may convince you too can be another skiing great on the ski slopes just by imagining you are another famous French Olympian like Claude Killy.

Recalling that many falls can be avoided cognitively. THINK. AVOID. Remember, you are no longer in your mid-30s. But preventive techniques like building stronger legs doing squats on the Bosu ball will help you avoid future mishaps and falls. Stints on the ball can be as vital for you as it has been for me. Mastering the manoeuvres on it I have described helped correct my bout with vertigo, benign paroxysmal vertigo, much more than the Epley manoeuvre,

Shoulder strengthening is vital to enhance function while eliminating pain. I remain sceptical that shoulder surgery is for everyone. Rotator cuff surgery seems like overkill when I see some poor soul with a shoulder immobiliser for months after surgery. If you do not have a full tear or multiple tears, why not try strengthening alternative supporting muscles like the deltoid, the thin shoulder muscle that flays around the head of the humerus?

Try using an over-the-head pulley, bringing each arm up from the horizontal to vertical allowing the opposite arm to provide resistance as it is pulled up. I described the value of this technique to stretch out weak rotator cuff muscles in the stretching chapter. Biceps curls and triceps extensions with 5 to 10 pounds is another effective method to add strength and ease pain in a challenged shoulder. Strengthen muscles around diarthrodial joints like the knee and elbow, or ball-in-socket joints like the shoulder or hip.

Strengthening your gluteals, Maximus, Medius, and Minimus, will help encroaching proximal muscle weakness such as getting up from the dining room chair or getting up after falling to the floor. Strong gluteals are also vital for gait and balance. Losing muscle mass especially of your butt muscles can present other mundane challenges as holding your pants up. Work those gluteals.

Now, let us get into the specifics.

Essentials of a Great Strength Program:

Keep it light. Keep it fun. Mix it up. Be spontaneous, but be careful not to overdo it. Exercise savants recommend three to four strength training sessions weekly. With plenty of time on your hands after retirement, fitting a strength training program into your schedule can be easier. Remember, the YMCA system has reciprocity. So, if you're on the road visiting one of your grandchildren in another state, the "Y" can be the way to go. I'm an outdoor quick-change artist. Bring your gym togs along. Also, remember to bring a dry shirt and socks. No sense in getting chilled due to a wet shirt. In doubt how to begin? The American College of Sports Medicine recommends and has a list of qualified exercise specialists. No excuses please! More is not better? Doing is better.

Exercise machines like the Nautilus prototype, unlike free weights, reduce the chance of exercising in the wrong way. Isokinetic exercise on machines isolates specific muscle groups with adjustable and quantifiable amounts of resistance followed by a controlled relaxation phase. Breathing in with exertion and breath out on the release. Avoid a ballistic release phase to avoid injury. On the road, bring along exercise tubing available at any athletic store as an alternative way to maintain muscles tone.

Specific Strength Training Techniques

- **Pyramid Type** – My technique is to start a lift technique with a weight or number on a machine just at a weight where I am feeling a challenge, then go up a notch with each set so that by the end of my third set, I can feel the burn but not pain.
- **Heavy-to-light** – Not my choice. I prefer upping the weight with each set as above.
- **Lift-Rest-Lift** – Begin with what you have determined has been the maximum weight you can lift. Rest. Repeat until the point you can go no further. Do not minimise your ability.
- **Compound Technique** – Mix it up: combine a biceps curl with a press combined with active rest between both combined techniques.
- **Reps and Sets** – Try 10 to 15 repetitions ("Reps") with either a specific challenging weight or by increasing 5 to 10 pounds with each set in a pyramid fashion and doing as many sets as work for you.
- **Cheater** – An example is a biceps curl by going straight down, dropping your arms toward your feet with your arms fully extended. Beginning with a comfortable weight start the curl with a bump from your quadriceps. Then, let your biceps takes over for the full curl.

For those of you with a weaker upper body for the pullup, begin by standing on a loop at the bottom of bungee cord attached to the support bar and begin your lift with a bounce making it easier to reach the bar with your chin. If an exercise partner is nearby, have him give your legs a bear hug and initiate a biceps curl against your supported weight. I had my Nordic Ski Team – especially the gals – use the foot-in-the bungee technique to bypass a weaker upper body

- **The Split Technique** – Split training areas of your body.
- Group 1 – Monday, Wednesday, Friday for your legs, back and trunk (core).
- Group 2 – Tues, Thurs, Sat, do your chest, shoulders, and back. This regimen works well for the body builders.
- **Peripheral** – Balance one exercise far removed from another body part to avoid over fatiguing either; for example, do a calf lift and then move on to a bench press. This technique is faster and is useful for someone with a time restraint.
- **Circuit training** – This program enhances aerobic endurance. With this modality you can do lighter weights while shortening your rest period. By doing so, and as you push it, you can combine an aerobic with an anaerobic work-out.
- **Super Circuit** – This technique is the basis of a Jillian Michaels program. Integrating an aerobic warmup comprised of a 30 second to a minute of demanding aerobic activity – jumping jacks, running in place, aerobic dancing, to elevate your heart rate to a Level 3–4 intensity (defined as a moderate to high intensity workout). Then, intersperse the

fun with a combination of light weights or resistance exercises such as push-ups, sit-ups, or crunches. No time to rest. It's back to aerobic moves turning into level four intensity that morphs to an anaerobic level.

- **Cardiovascular Fitness Pyramid** More information on fitness training in the Aerobic chapter to come.

Level 5 – Red Zone (90–100% of your maximal heart rate).
Level 4 – Anaerobic Zone (90–100% of your maximal heart rate).
Level 3 – Aerobic Zone (70–85% of your maximal heart rate).
Level 2 – Healthy Heart Zone (50–70% of your maximal heart rate).
Level 1 – Weight Management Zone (40–50% of your maximum heart rate)

- Michael's program intersperses lighter weights (curls, squats), at higher reps for alternating muscle groups. She advocates this approach to increase lean muscle mass, maintain flexibility, and develop more strength while all the while stretching before and after her super circuit.

Weight Training Exercises

- **Biceps** – "Curls for the girls:" either standing or lying. Remember gentle does it, especially on the relaxation phase as you lower the bar. Alternatively, using a machine insures you will engage a controlled lowering of the weight. Inhale on the lift, exhale on the return down.
- another technique is lying on your back and curling the free weights up and toward your body.

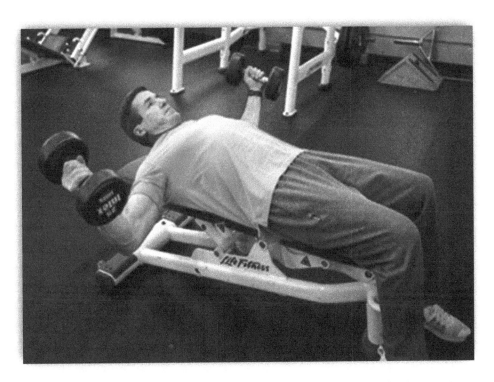

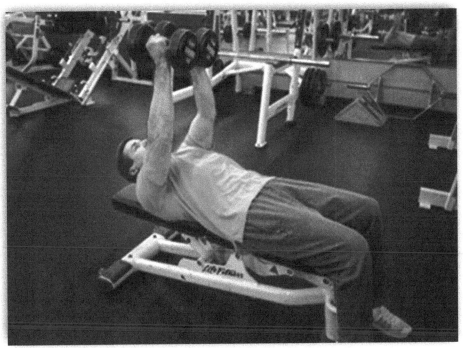

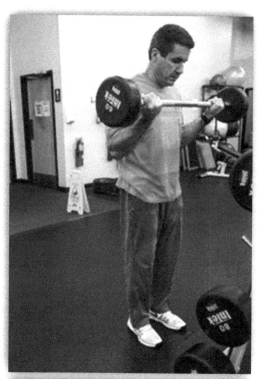

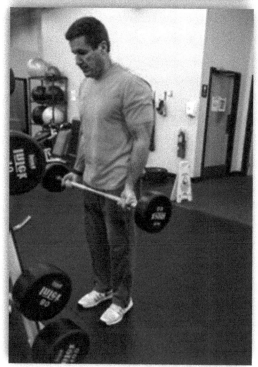

The Plank – Now, here's a way to strengthen almost every muscle on your chassis, by that I mean the nuts and bolts of your body.

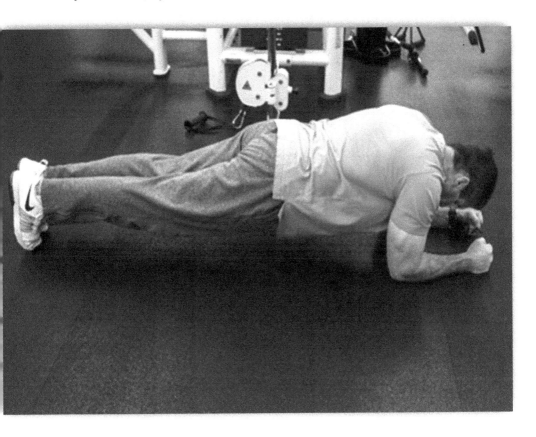

- This technique is why yoga is so good for you – either down on your elbows or up on hands keeping elbows straight.

Remember to continue breathing as you tense those triceps, long muscles of your back, and here's where the tires hit the road. YOUR CORE! You are also throwing in the quads and calves.

Triceps – Keep it nice and comfortable. Keep one knee on the weight bench and the opposite outstretched arm on the bench while lifting your arm holding the weight from a 45-degree angle to your body. Let it rip slowly and not ballistically as you lift your forearm back into extension. Breathe in on the extension and out on relaxation back to the original 45 degree angle, poling will now be your strongest suit.

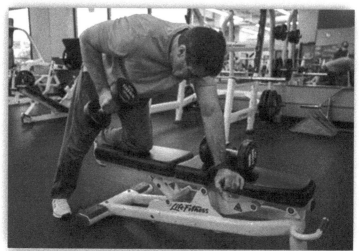

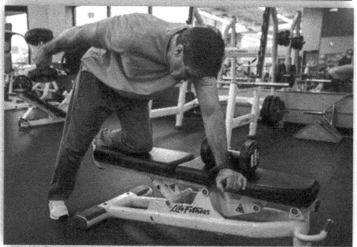

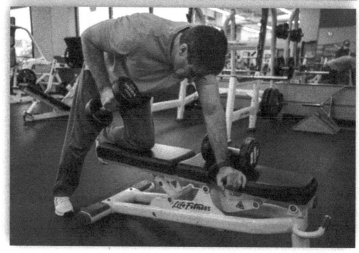

Now you've made headway strengthening both your biceps and triceps muscles so important in lifting that bag of leaves or your robust grandson. If you're a cross country skier, poling will now be a cinch.

Your pectoralis on your chest and the long muscles on your back like this cable pulldown exercise.

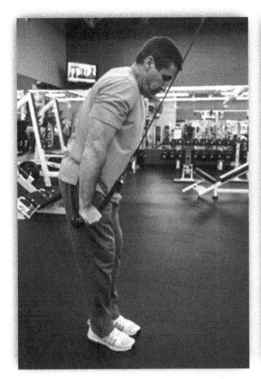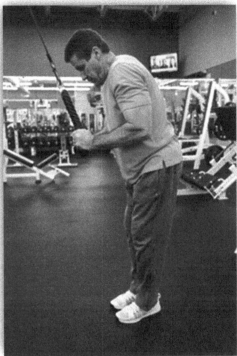

Cable Pull Downs- can also offer some extras to the triceps exercises described above, but especially strengthening your "pecs" and long muscles of your back, the latissimus dorsalis muscles. Remember, breath in when you pull down and out as you return to the start position.

Bench Press – For your "Pecs", deltoids, and further arm strengthening of your triceps, lie on a weight bench for less strain for your back, and bringing in more for the abdominals.

- Grasp the Weights. Inhale as you lift. Exhale as you return the weights to your shoulders. Take care, this is one exercise when it is essential to have a spotter.

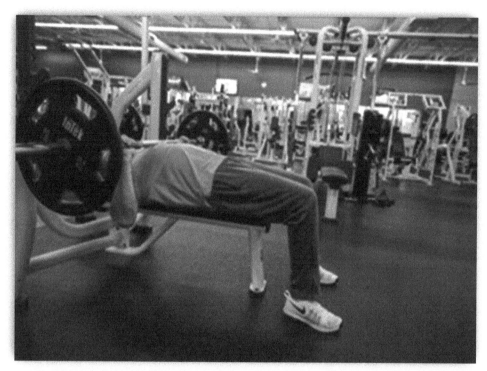

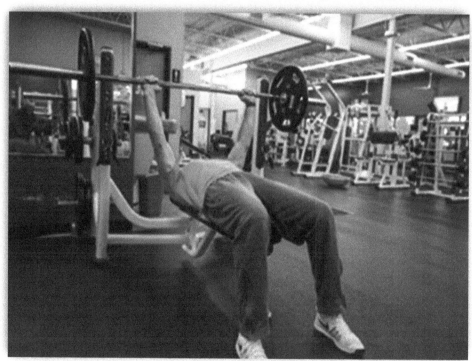

- **Half Squats** – For your "glutes," hamstrings, "quads," and your erector spinae –the little muscles that, with the latissimus dorsalis, support your lower back. These muscles can be injured more easily when lifting incorrectly or going gonzo to set a personal record how much weight you think you can lift. Forget it!. Remember. Go low and slow for starters. Consider wearing a lifting belt. Take your choice. You can use either free weights sitting or standing, or a squat machine that may be easier on your back as it may control the relaxation phase better. Note, doing the same exercise on a machine but recumbent may be better on your back.

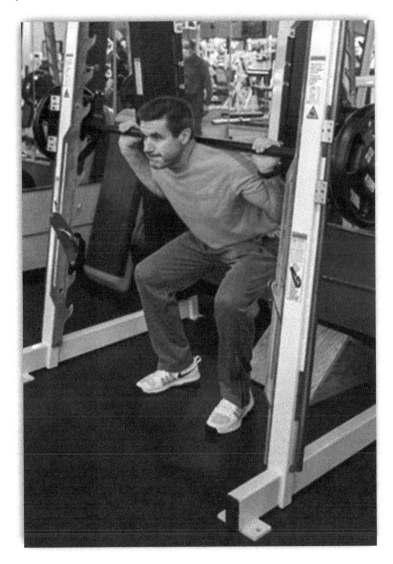

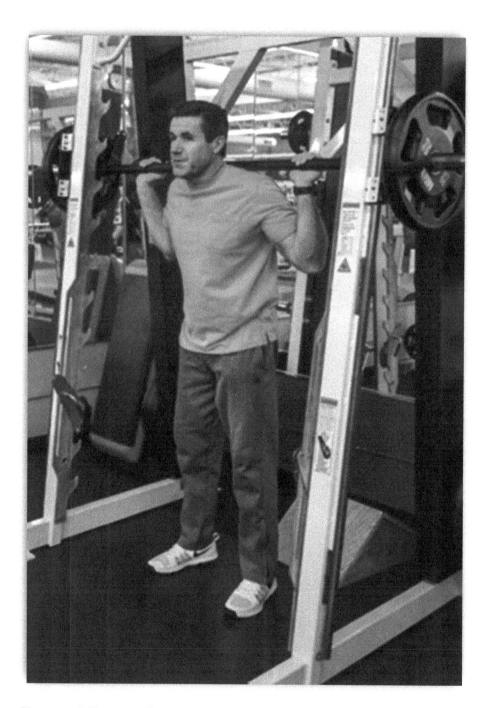

Clean and Press – For your erector spinae, "gluts", hamstrings, "traps", deltoids, triceps, and serratus anterior – also called the "big-swing muscle". This muscle group pulls your scapula around and holds it to the rib cage. Also, it is important in throwing a punch.

How to – With the weights on the floor and your, feet wide apart, grip the bar and slowly bring the weight up to your waist as you inhale, exhaling while bringing the weight back to the floor. As noted, the lifter, Doug Hagerty, skips the final clean and jerk part of the lift only bringing the bar up to his waist as he straightens up his back. This manoeuvre is terrific for the quads and all the muscles, small and large, of the back that further strengthen your core.

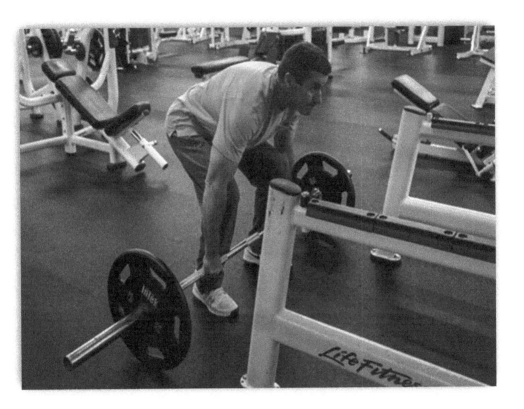

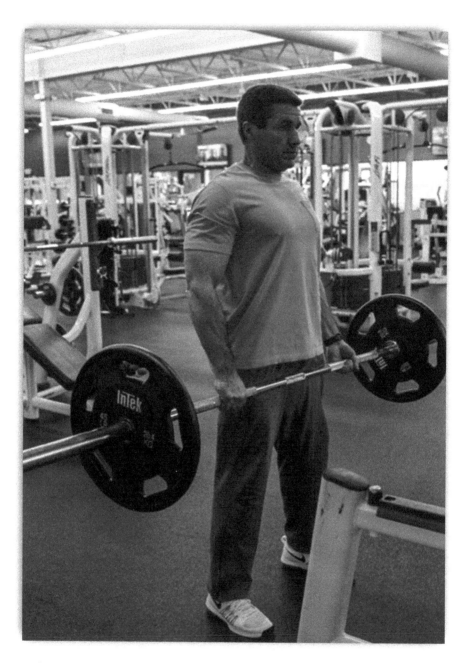

Alternately and not pictured is the clean and jerk that is overkill and can be rough on the shoulders. If you want to do it, here's how and as with most exercises strengthening back muscles described here, a weight belt is a good idea. With a graceful quick snap while inhaling bring the bar up under your chin. Rest for a split second before the most dramatic lift of them all as you raise both arms raised in a powerful victory salute capped by the bar bell. Success! Now, carefully bring the weights down to the mat but without a bang.

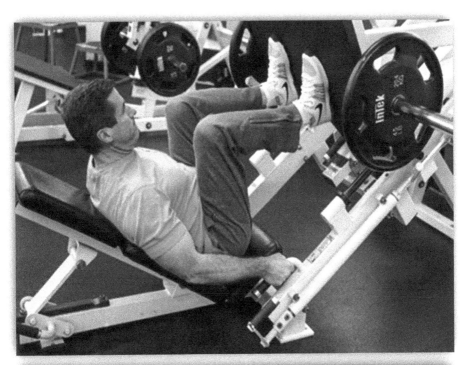

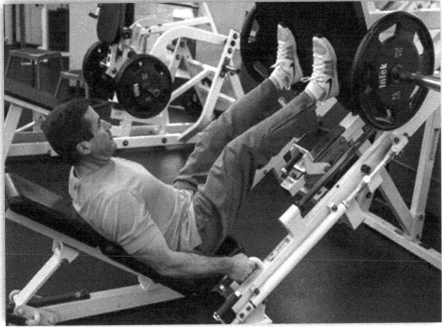

Calf Lifts – The gastrocnemius and soleus funnel down into that rascal, the Achilles tendon. You can stand with your toes on any step or board and rest a reasonable weight on the bar sitting on your shoulders as you raise and lower your body.

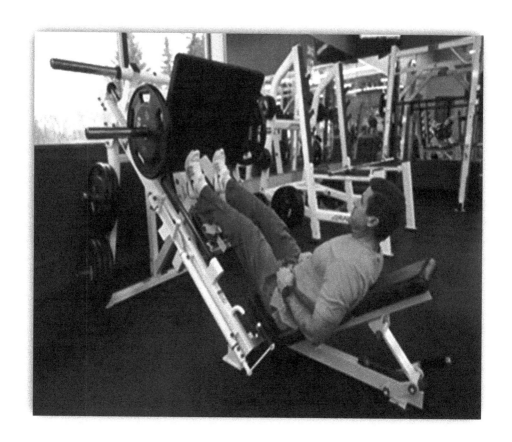

This time just lift the weights as you stand up on your toes on the platform either standing or recumbent pressing against a comfortable weight against the ball of your foot as you extend your legs flexing your toes and lighter weights with more repeats is safer on the Achilles tendon. Then, relax as your legs return as you release your ankle flexion while breathing out.

Don't forget to breath even though you're working the bottom part of your body. This exercise is an excellent way to strengthen your calves. Like stretching described earlier, this exercise is an excellent way to avoid injuring your Achilles tendon.

Dips – Enhances triceps again; the deltoids streaming over your shoulders; chest muscles, the pectoralis major, and minor; and the latissimus dorsi, those long muscle that run all along the length of your back along the spine to support your back; keep it straight, strong, and comfortable while you are standing or lifting.

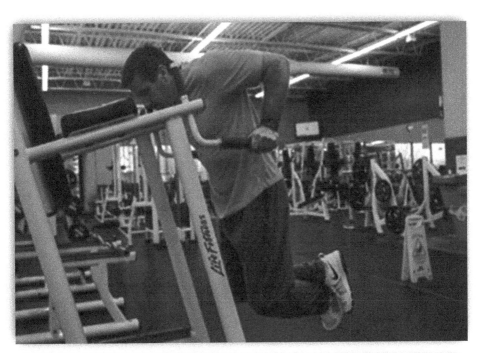

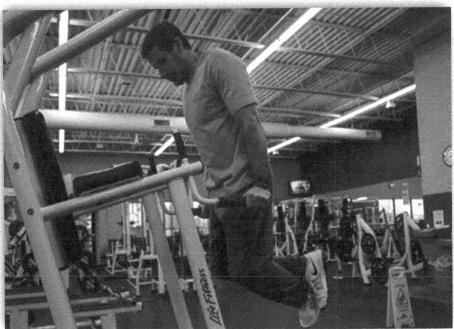

How to – Grip the parallel bars, palms down. Now, let yourself down while exhaling. Then on an inhale, bring your body up again. That is the hard part.

Back Extensions - A more difficult challenge is comfortably lowering your upper body folding at the waist over a supporting bar, your lower body held in place by a bar behind your heels.

Go slowly and if you want to further the challenge gradually upping a weight you can hold behind your neck. Exhale as you drop your upper body and inhale as you return to the lifted position.

Back Extensions enhance the erector spinae, hamstrings, gluteals (major, Medius, minor), the trapezoids, and rhomboids that hold your scapula in place and stabilize your shoulders.

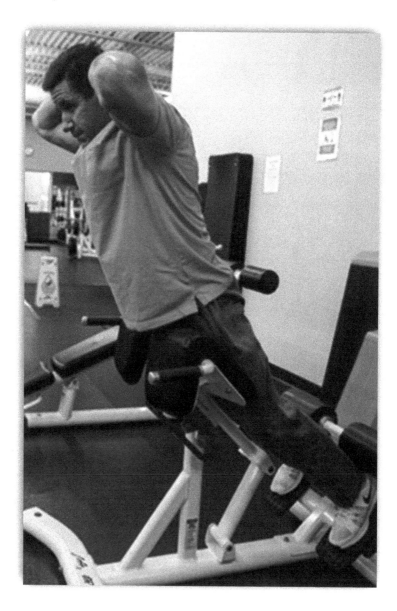

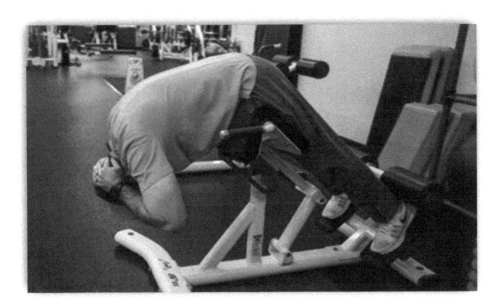

Incline sit-ups –
Strengthen your upper abdominal rectus muscle. You do not need to go all the way up from the board, but you can lie with your back to 45 degrees then lift as your muscles tighten as you then pull yourself up toward your feet. I prefer doing a crunch only partially lifting.

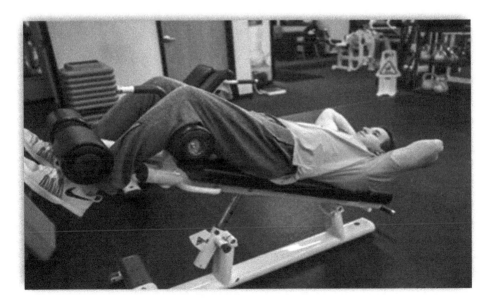

As with back extensions, I like to increase the weight of the barbell behind my neck between reps. As with any resistance exercise, it is important to tailor your program to any physical issues to avoid injury or pain. Remember to breath: inhale on the crunch, exhale as you slowly and comfortably lower your body.

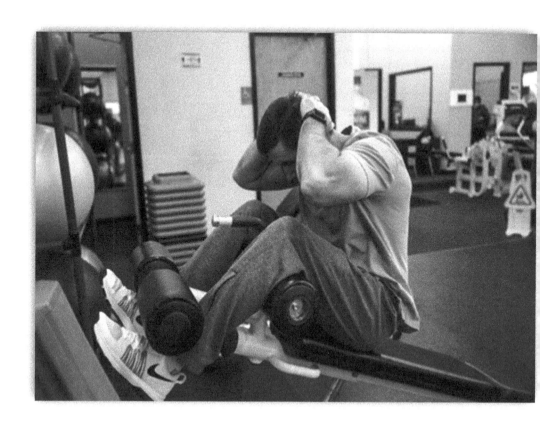

Leg lifts – Gets the lower abdominal recti muscles.

How to – Mount a platform resting the back of your forearm while holding a short vertical pommel. Lower your legs and as you do, exhale.
Breathe in as you lift your legs to the horizontal exhale as you slowly lower your legs.

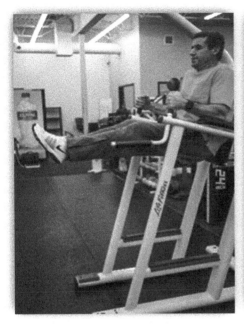 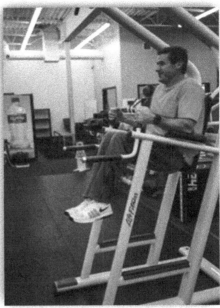

Lateral Pulldowns – Enhances your latissimus dorsi, teres major, rhomboids, and biceps.

How to – Sit on the seat of the pulldown machine, holding the bar above your head. Pull down either in front of your chin or down behind your head onto your shoulders.

All rules apply about breathing and staying slow and steady but not ballistic. Inhale pulling down and exhaling as you let the bar glide back up.

Thigh adductors and Extenders – Great for Your quadriceps, thigh and hip adductors (gracilis, obturator externus, adductor longus, brevis, and magnus); or on the abduction, and your hip abductors (piriformis, superior gemellus, tensor fascia lata, sartorius, gluteus Medius, and minimus). So much for anatomy.

How to – I advise care especially on the adduction part of the drill; that is, when you bring your thighs together that you avoid any groin muscle or tendon overuse or tear. When you perform this exercise with the pad on the inside for adduction or outside (abduction) of your thighs, do the standard breathing pattern. Inhale on adducting and abducting, respectively, then exhaling on the release.

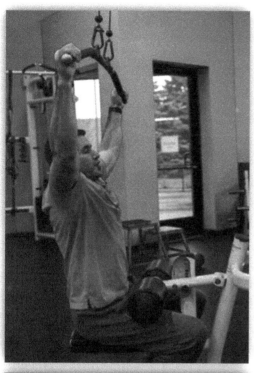 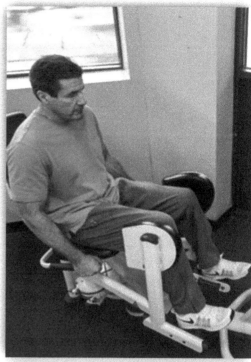

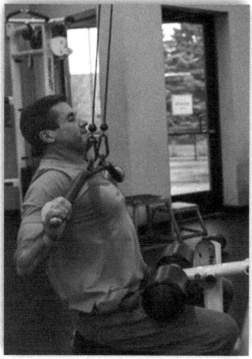 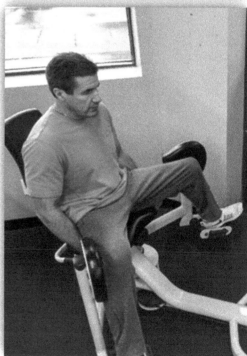

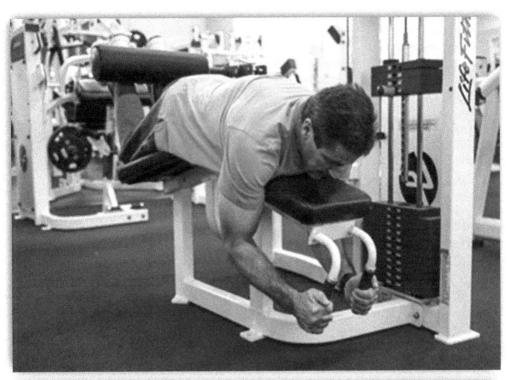

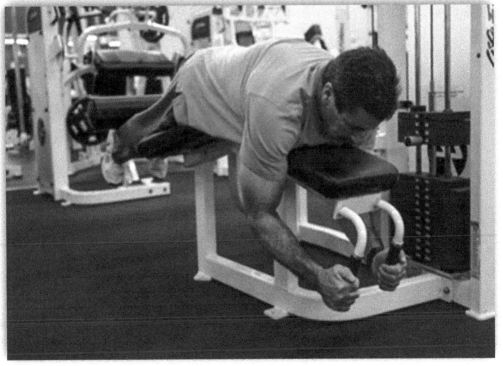

Quadriceps and Hamstring Curls

How to – the machines are self-explanatory It is important, especially with the hamstring curls, to start at a safe weight and avoid a ballistic release. Those hamstrings can be tricky devils.

Remember, our hamstrings are overpowered by the quadriceps. So, go low and slow increasing weights judiciously with each set.

My advice is to err on the conservative side until you have found the weight progression that is comfortable and safe for you.

Overall, with all the resistance exercises. If in doubt, ask for help from a knowledgeable friend or gym professional.

These strength training recipes are meant as an abbreviated guide. Try three sets of 10 repetitions for starters for the circuit described above and whatever weight changing technique you find best for yourself. There are plenty of You Tube videos available to flesh out a more detailed recipe. This short guide for developing and maintaining strength is designed to ignite a fire under your butt. JUST GET GOING heeding the proverb, "Use it or lose it!" These are exercises that can delay an inevitable decrease in the strength and power of muscles that are devolving as we age. Reassuring information such as these empowering exercises will slow down or, even better, stabilize and, best yet, revitalize strength, power, and joy derived from the play of fitness. In lieu of the current pandemic, video workouts of any kind may be the new hybrid of the future.

Chapter 13
Aerobics Exercise

The ACSM recommends exercising aerobically with three, four, or more thirty-minute workouts a day to a sweat plus two to three strength sessions a week. Doing so can be a sure-fire escape from stress. A predominance of genetically determined slow-twitch muscle fibres favour endurance before speed. Long slow workouts enhance endurance also by increasing oxygenating peripheral capillaries. A heart monitor can ensure you're always in an effective training zone. Take a day or two of active easy rest days a week. Experience fitness and fun. Throw in bursts of high intensity exercise regardless of heart or lung issues. But, first, if you have risk factors, check with your physician first. Forget the "No pain, no gain" myth. Make it pleasurable, convenient, and consistent. Unsure? Hire a trainer. If she or he is good marry her/him!

"Many studies show that depressed patients who stick to a regimen of aerobic exercise improve as much as those treated with medicine."
– Andrew Weil, M.D.
Author, *Spontaneous Healing* (1995)

Our older set (Careful, now, do not say "old") enter the slower, take-longer category. The "sex" chapter suggests there are some advantages for taking longer. As we age, we depend more on slow-twitch muscle fibres. They have greater oxygen carrying capacity and enhance endurance (aerobic) capacity, and are great for long, slow activities. For younger sprinters, fast-twitch fibres predominate for the bursts of speed of an anaerobic 100-yard dash or split-second long jump. If you are competitive and inclined, consider masters' competition.

Hatfield and Krotee explain why one or another athlete is faster at either the short or long distance. They explain is that "The ratio of fast-twitch to slow-twitch fibres is genetically determined and cannot change by training."

There is a physiological difference between the two types of fibres – fast-twitch fibres depend on high-energy compounds.... Slow twitch fibres are enhanced by the size and number of energy units. Endurance exercise is the successful marriage of anaerobic and aerobic pathways of metabolism with the effectiveness of slow-twitch fibres increasing with age. Training that incorporates long slow distance (LSD) increases capillarisation that feeds oxygenated blood to slow-twitch fibres. This concept explains why we as older athletes can still excel in endurance activities.

Adhere to a schedule if you can. Knowing you have a Barre or Pilates class at 7:30 helps make sleeping in less likely. For men over 60, health insurance supports prevention with programs like Silver and Fit or Silver Sneakers that are available through most health plans. Exercising, communal or solitary is a personal preference. Make sweating a regular activity. Patiently increase the intensity of your work-out. Too many New Year's Day resolutions start too hard, lead to injuries, or hurt so much the day afterward, that a convert calls it quits. They lose the desire to continue a good thing. But do not let that be you. Do not overdo it. Do it!

- Barre derived from the barre discipline in classic dance, safely combines dynamic-active stretches, light weights, and yoga. Those who advocate Barre enthusiasts explain that it increases flexibility, lengthens muscles, and makes their bodies stronger and more graceful.
- The Pilates Method, started in late 20th century and continuing to the present, uses special exercises on apparatuses – the Universal Reformer, the Cadillac, and the Chair –to strengthen the health of the human mind and body. Like yoga, breathing is central to this discipline, engages the mind and, unlike isometrics on machines, focuses on specific muscle engagement and core stabilisation.

The American College of Sports Medicine (ACSM) addresses the challenge how much exercise is good and when does it become counterproductive. ACSM advocates three to four aerobic days plus two to three strength days with a few days off a week. I prefer my own alternate day routine starting with an aerobic warmup like a short run followed by a circuit on the machines, barbells, or backyard exercises like push-ups, pull-ups, a roller board described earlier, incline crunches, and leg lifts on an incline. My tired muscles thank me on my rest days. I do longer and easier workouts like hikes, bike rides or laps in the pool on my rest days. Such down days' supply active rest.

Mixing up your program with biking, hiking, roller blading, or swimming is another way to mobilise a different set of muscles on alternate days, and not get bored doing the same old thing day after day. I am less worried about a hodgepodge workout including intervals, long slow distance, weightlifting, or barre than about not exercising at all. I try not to be obsessive and, to that end, do not keep exercise logs. Stick as best you can to an exercise schedule and be circumspect to allow for active rest days. Save the weekends to spend with your partner. I do and it works wonders for our relationship.

Jogging, the successful aerobic exercise – a form of trotting or running at a slow or leisurely pace, was promoted by New Zealand coach, Arthur Lydiard in 1962. It was as much about aerobic exercise as fitness and sociability. Running, biking, cross-country skiing. swimming, dancing, hiking, accomplish a similar goal. Join a group as I have described that combines a sport with a convivial post exercise coffee and scones. Sadly, speed or intensity may not increase your lifespan. By improving strength, aerobic fitness, and agility you can attain greater exercise tolerance and, let's hope, an improved quality of life. I love the expression, "I want to grow older younger." "Developing fitness promotes greater endurance capacity and the love and enjoyment of everyday life" so says Norwegian super star, Sven Edvinson Salje, "Livet skal vaera en gave, Life is a gift."

How Much Is Too Much?

Some form of aerobic cardiac exercise at 65 to 85% of your V0$_2$max, the maximum volume of oxygen you can use exercising as hard as you can, is ideal Approaching your V0$_2$ max, but no higher than Level 3 – while you can still chat with your training partner – does a world of good regardless of whether you are competitive or just aiming for fitness. Exercise intensity is also based on METS or how much energy your body is able to use during exercise. One MET equals3.5 millilitres of oxygen divided by how much you weigh in kilograms times a minute—or while just sitting around). Dr Ken Cooper, who wrote *Aerobics* in 1968, designed a simple fitness test that includes a 12-minute run. But, just starts by walking 10,000 steps a day to maintain fitness. That is what my partner, Nada, strives for every day with her Smart Health watch.

Strive for three aerobic sessions a week or more if you want of at least 30 minutes each ideally to a sweat at 65–75% of your maximal heart rate (220-age). You do not have to suffer. Attaining this level is well below your anaerobic threshold – when painful lactic acid saturates your muscles, and they just won't go any further. This is when you wonder if you are getting water boarded. Exercise is most effective in the comfort zone – well below your anaerobic threshold. A good reference point is that an exercise stress test (GXT) only reaches 85% of your calculated maximal heart rate and, and is well within the safety zone while effectively assessing your cardiac status.

Rules For Success?

1) **Frequency** – Keep exercising regular to reinforce a good habit. Mix it up. Alternate hard with easy workout days, and take it easy the day after hard or longer activity.
2) **Duration** – Sports experts suggest aerobics several times a week (three to five) for as little as 30 minutes and, preferably, to a sweat.
3) **Intensity** – Follow the gold standard to calculate maximal heart rate: Count your pulse for 10 seconds and multiply by 6 to measure how your workout relates to your calculated maximal heart rate. How hard you work determines how many calories you burn, how quickly you build endurance, and whether you are getting the absolute most out of your exercise time.

Level 1: 50-60% (light) of maximal heart rate (MHR). Weight management level and a light exercise like walking. Level 1 burns carbohydrates first, then fat. Measured by METs-- the ratio of your working metabolic rate relative to your resting metabolic rate, is the rate

of energy expanded per unit time. This level should be thirty minutes or more, three to four times a week. Do not forget those strength workouts!

Level 2: 60-70% of your MHR (Slow and steady). This level builds endurance by increasing muscle capillaries: Here again follow the 30 minute rule three or four times a week is the ticket. Generally less than three METS.

Level 3: 70-80% of MHR (Getting harder but talking still). Improves aerobic fitness and muscle strength: 30-40minutes, or more three to four times a week. With longer exercise times you will deplete glycogen stores. This level is 3 to six METS.

Level 4: 80-90% of MHR is also called The Red Zone. (This is when you cannot carry on a conversation). Throw in bursts for a few seconds up to a minute of HIIT. Intervals of HIIT increase your VO_2 $_{MAX}$-especially part of sprints for the high-performance athletes among you. You're hitting your lactate threshold. Levels 4 and 5 greater than 6 METS.

Level 5: 90-100% of MHR. Anaerobic metabolism Especially for the higher performance athlete and key to effective the starts, passing, and the finish of races. This level is how you can boost your lactate levels and is when your muscles really begin to hurt and not for the faint of heart.

One simple way to know you are getting past a level three work-out is that once you enter level four you are no longer able to hold a conversation with your running best buddy. When you are gasping for breath and unable to continue sad tales about a bad day at the office, ups and downs with your wife, or dealing with an errant kid, you are closing in on your anaerobic threshold. Cut back a notch to level three so you can resume your tales of woe.

Amazing older athlete, Dr Bill Andberg, whose mantra was, "Live long and die young," got the moniker, "The Gray Ghost", after he was seen running through a cemetery one night in a gray sweat suit." Dr. Bill" began running at 60 and he advocated "red lining"; that is, up and over your anaerobic threshold. It worked...for him, anyway. Among his many running accomplishments, Andberg, a veterinarian, in 1968, at the first National Masters Track Championships took gold in the marathon in his age group. At Toronto in 1975, he won gold again in the over 60 age group in both the 1500 and 3000 metre races. Andberg's high-end successful training sounds a bit like Jane Brody's high intensity interval workouts(HIIT). Dick Beardsley tells how he can remember every mile of his marathons. Beardsley said, "I can remember when I started, when I finished, and when I vomited." Even victors like Dr Andberg and Beardsley feel the pain but sustain hard training.

Exercise specialist, Ken McAlpine describes how to exercise harder but suffer less. He advocates exercising at a higher heart rate. Many athletes advocate a heart monitor to monitor that they stay in the best training zone. The onetime house painter and eponymous master's cross-country ski world champion, Bjorn Lasserud, who, faced with little free time, described his workout as hard, harder, and hardest. How successful you can be with this approach is how hard you train, the true grit of Bjorn but often more about the parents we did not choose. He conquered alcoholism at 40, and raced sober until his knees went out in his early 80s. Bjorn was always good for a good laugh and helped many aspiring athletes love their sport and achieve their potential.

Is it possible to attain fitness without gonzo high-intensity workouts? Yes. There is, however, the saying in the ski racing world that "training slow means racing slow". If you want the competitive edge, you best summon balls-to-the-walls, high-intensity training. But enough about competition. This book is about maintaining and staying. Oh, I almost forgot – most of all – having fun.

Many endurance athletes strap on a heart monitor programmed to later download a workout. By doing so, you can monitor what is too little or too much exercise intensity. A heart monitor can log work-out time, terrain, levels of intensity, as well as time spent at different altitude, and the topography of your work-out. A heart monitor follows your heart rate and, by signalling you, can help you back off a bit to re-enter an effective exercise zone.

Good news: an over-60 athlete can judiciously train at levels three and four but preferably at the latter, for limited periods of time. Integrating your exercise program with high intensity interval training (HIIT) activities can also improve cardiac function for the healthy as well as someone with heart disease, COPD, or other chronic illnesses. Active rest becomes more important with age. Imagine exercise as an escape and relaxation counterpoint to work and stress.

Using a monitor resembles phase three cardiac rehabilitation programs that monitor post "MI" patients preventing them from taking cardiac risks due to excessive levels of exercise. In cardiac rehab, an exercise monitor can detect dangerous rhythms during exercise or immediately afterward.

I find a chest monitor too constraining and just check my pulse at the top of a long or challenging hill. Some athletes chose to work with a trainer who can design their exercise program. Some keep training logs. Do whatever works for you. Remember, what you choose should not hurt, and you should like doing it. Where you exercise should be convenient, and, primarily, let it be fun.

You can learn a great deal about your body by simply checking your pulse when you first wake up. Although there are individual variations, a pulse for most over 100, tachycardia, suggests you may be overtraining, you are tired, possibly getting sick, or on an over-the-counter medication such as a cold remedy containing pseudoephedrine(Sudafed) or phenylephrine(Sudafed PE). Take the day or week off. A pulse of sixty or less, bradycardia, is usual among endurance athletes. When I landed in the ER with chest pain a few years after two stents imagining it was angina, I could see the concern on the face of the ER doc since my pulse was forty. Thinking I might be in a dangerous rhythm, the crew was getting ready to grab the paddles.

'Hey, hey, wait a minute. Are any of you an athletes?' I asked her.

I got an affirmative from the young and strongly built ER physician. I grabbed the still-warm EKG strip from the technician behind me, took a quick look, and, waving it, said confidently.

'It's just a slow rate. I am an endurance athlete!'

They were worried that I might be in a two to one heart block when upper atrial beats do not translate into an effective ventricular contraction. There are several other possibilities for someone with a pulse as low as mine. I could be taking a beta-blocker like Inderal (propranolol) or Lopressor (metoprolol) to lower my blood pressure that also lowers heart rate.

Train Alone or With a Partner or Group?

Generally, I like to exercise and train alone. For others, there can be an element of solidarity and who enjoy the camaraderie of other weightlifters grunting and groaning, as they try to dead lift or squat their personal best. Some prefer structured programs available at most gyms ranging from Pilates, yoga, the ballet-inspired barre, or a marathon training program with the American Lung Association. The latter has encouraged many to complete their first marathon.

One friend runs a regular Saturday hike or bike capped by a destination coffee house for plenty of visiting accompanied by coffee and treats. Many in the retirement set look for like-minded training friends for an early morning of biking, skiing, or in-line skating.

Mixing up your exercise regimen is a helpful way to avoid overuse issues. What has occurred for me, trying to break the doldrums with longer or harder workout sessions is producing lots of lactate. I feel zapped and can become short-tempered. Some, unfortunately may wake up with a rapid pulse, unexplained fatigue, or depression. Such physical and emotional lability can be over training or, worse yet, burnout. It can sneak up on you. I advise starting slowly as you begin a new exercise regimen. More may not be better. Your body can play tricks when an overachiever has lost control and fails to cut back. So, listen to your body. It often knows what your head may not understand.

Alternative forms of great non-impact aerobic exercise like swimming may not protect as well as impact exercise like running against osteoporosis. Consider the Stairmaster or a low-impact aerobics step program. As a society, we are in big trouble. Seventy% of adults aged 20 and over are overweight. Ideal body mass index, (BMI) is 18.5–25; whereas 25-29.9 is overweight. Over 30 is obese. BMI is your height in inches (centimetres) divided by your weight in pounds (kilograms). So, get out there and challenge the statistics! At least change yours!

I have tried them all; heart monitors, weight vests, intervals on my bike, roller blades, roller-skiing up and down a pot-holed parkway, or running any hills I can find. I strive for to 65–85% of my VO_2 max for most of my exercising. My partner, Nada, and I take hikes an enjoyable hour and one-half to 3 or 4 hours while vacationing off the Lake Superior Hiking Trail overlooking a pristine Lake Superior or at a local county park. I can surreptitiously ramp it up by taking plyometric jumps behind Nada, folding in speed bursts. These walks include healing talks, the sure cure for any bumps in the road of our relationship. It's cheaper and more effective than marital counselling.

In these days of errant drivers on their cell phones, staying off the roads may be a good idea. Bringing a friend alongside can support your commitment to regular exercise. It's worth knowing that the largest contingent to participate in World Masters Cross Country Ski Championships are the over 60 set. We just have more discretionary money and time to train and compete. My 80-year-old friend, Odd, joins a supervised training group as the token older person. He, starts on a cold winter's day at 6:30 am at a trail when the temperature can be a good zero degrees or colder Brrrrh! But, he loves it and is admired for his perseverance despite his age.

Odd's choice is much cheaper than a psychiatrist and possibly just as good as group therapy. He prides himself as being the oldest athlete in training. It works for Odd who won several gold or bronze medals in the 2022 World Cross Country Ski Championships at Canmore, Canada. Plenty of those who are still cursed to get to work by eight are on the trails for their very early morning workout with a head lamp by 5:30. Many like exercising in tune with their best diurnal rhythm. I have always been an exercise opportunist, grabbing any window of opportunity, but I usually like to get at it first thing in the morning. You are the one who knows what time is best for your mind and body. This decision is an individual thing.

In *Dr D's Handbook*, I explained that cortisol and testosterone peak at 4 a.m. Phylogenetically, such a hormonal burst is getting you ready to hunt the woolly mammoth or at least escape from one. We can also take advantage of high levels of serotonin and testosterone for a good shot on the day by exercising early. I have a recollection when I was the occupational health physician for a local hospital, and – instead of lunching in the doctor's lounge, jumped into running gear and burst out the clinic doors to join my running analyst friend, a serious runner and psychiatrist. Running the city streets and lakes, I was always at the upper edge of Level 3 choosing breathing over therapy. After a quick sponge bath, I was back seeing patients… a wonderful memory.

An ageless Olympic and World Cup gold medallist in the 4X10 relay at the Winter Olympics in Salt Lake City.), Norwegian cross country ski icon, Anders Aukland, happily delights in sharing his once secret training log. Now 50, he advises, "Train smart… not too much, not too little. Make good use of your time. Bike to work. Make it simple, not complicated. Train at home to save time, and adjust your training schedule to your family and life schedules. Progress is the driver. Think for yourself and find a training group. Set a goal and create a training plan that will help you reach your goal."

He adds, "Using a heart monitor. Well, that is your call. I prefer training unencumbered, finding my deepest thoughts while sweating. My mantra is always: "Listen to your body. Pick your coach or trainer well. Remember, the point of exercising or competing is to accomplish goals by having fun while challenging yourself. After all, your workouts are supposed to be escapes from stress, not contributing to it."

Find a trainer who can guide you without setting off alarms. A trainer should be objective and may just need to say, 'Relax. Take some time off.' Conversely, a trainer may push you where you never thought you could go – to the pain of a high intensity interval workout, or just say, "Take it easy, my friend". If you are ready to take a chance, even explore the benefits of red lining a time or two as my exercise friends, Bjorn and Dr. Bill Anders, have done.

Chapter 14
An Ounce of Prevention
When, Where and How

At 60, you are NOT "over-the-hill", this chapter is the "dos and don'ts" of exercise. Pick a physician who exercises. Dropout rates are significant; so, raise the bar low and slow as it feels good. If you are high risk, get a baseline electrocardiogram, a bike, treadmill, or echo stress test that, if suspicious, expect further tests such as a thallium radioactive study, a Cardiolite Stress Test, or the gold standard, the angiogram. Anticipate some sore muscles but, know when to back off. Drink plenty of water. Stretch before, during, after, and even while you exercise. If you are exercising below 32 degrees Fahrenheit. and that could be five months of the year as it can be in Minnesota, protect all exposed skin. Wear breathable, wicking, UV-protective clothing. Warning: hypothermia can occur above freezing.

"A doctor gave a man six months to live. The man couldn't pay his bill, so he gave him another six months."

– Henny Youngman

Many ask, "Should I have a stress test?" I would say, "Yes." If you are over 60 and if you have any of the hi-risk ingredients for a cardiac related problem such as Metabolic Syndrome: high blood pressure, diabetes, or just excess weight around your waist, you are at an increased risk for heart disease and stroke. You should also take into consideration other cardiac risk factors such as a history of smoking, high cholesterol, or triglyceride, or a strong family history for heart disease. My recommendation, as in *Dr D's Handbook for Men Over 40*, still applies. "Anyone over 60 who plans to push to their maximal heart rate deserves a baseline electrocardiogram, or with risk factors, a cardiac stress test."

There are plenty of options, including a simple stress test on a bike or treadmill, an echo stress test, or a thallium radioactive study. The thallium scan is a test that can also detect heart wall ischemia due to poor myocardial perfusion. It is called a nuclear stress test. It is done to show how well blood flows through the heart muscle. It also shows how well the heart muscle is pumping. For example, after a heart attack, it may be done to find areas of damaged heart muscle and, if someone is at a high risk exercising after a myocardial infarction, the test may be done during rest.

Another option, a Cardiolite Stress Test, demonstrates differences in the circulation of an isotope at rest and after exercise. Significant differences in these images may indicate a problem with the heart's blood supply relative to the coronary arteries. The gold standard is still coronary angiography to properly confirm abnormal or compromised coronary blood flow, cardiac output, the ejection fraction, and abnormal movement of cardiac muscle after a heart attack, or with ominous unstable angina.

Sports medicine experts determine higher levels of fitness based on your anaerobic threshold, also called the break point. Your VO2max is when lactic acid, the breakdown product of muscle oxidation, begins metabolising glucose less efficiently. Lactic acid accumulation is what makes our muscles hurt. Consistent exercising to the four to five levels elevates our anaerobic threshold Levels are different in everyone who exercises hard. Also, the VO2max has a lot to do with the parents you did not choose. Who says life is fair?

So, when are overdoing it? In *Dr D's Handbook* I listed two categories of overdoing it.

- **Immediate signs and symptoms**-include chest pain that could be angina, light-headedness, confusion, nausea, vomiting, unexplained leg pain or cramps, difficulty breathing, wheezing, inappropriately slow (Bradycardia=pulse <60 beats per minute) or fast heart rate (tachycardia= pulse > 100bpm), or a decrease in systolic blood pressure lower than 100 or diastolic blood pressure less than 60 while exercising.
- **Delayed signs and symptoms** – those lasting longer than 24 hours such as prolonged fatigue, insomnia, weight gain, leg swelling, difficulty breathing while exercising or while lying flat, or a persistent rapid heart rate.

Clearly, responding quickly to the described immediate symptoms rather than letting them progress into an irreversible meltdown is a necessity to avoid morphing into a more serious and potentially incapacitating injury. If you are concerned if it is safe for you to saddle up and start exercising, locate a physician who understands sports health. Choose one who will not pigeonhole you into an "over-the-hill" category.

It took several attempts locating sound medical advice for a painful arthritic big toe that led to successful surgery by an open-minded orthopaedist. He understood that a 70+-year-old old athlete like me would benefit from limited corrective surgery for bone spurs that was hindering my toe motion for hill bounding, hiking with Nada, or training and competing in upcoming ski marathons. Based on my desire to continue training and racing, he advised a less limiting surgery allowing mobility rather than fusing the toe joints

There is the bad but illustrative joke of the senior who goes to the doctor's office seeking advice and therapy for a painful left knee.

"You're over seventy", his doctor says. "Of course, you are bound to feel some pain".

Our graying senior warrior replies, "I know, doctor, but my right knee is also over 70 and IT doesn't hurt".

Find a physician who is a kindred spirit and understands how a senior athlete—himself included—wants and can stay fit into his 80s even 90s.

Take realistic precautions. When you head out on the trail for several hours, attach personal identification to your shoes, ski poles, or bike. Wear a wrist alert device if you have diabetes, pulmonary issues, or a history of heart disease. Use good judgment when it is too hot, too cold, or too humid. Adapt your exercise to weather demands. Carry a water bottle. Remember to drink water or a readily absorbable sports drink before, during, and after vigorous exercise. Drink a cup of fluid every 20 minutes while strenuously exercising regardless whether it is cold or warm out. In cold weather you are equally susceptible to dehydration as in warm weather. Water is perfect for exercise less than 30 minutes.

The next day after an extremely hard or long workout, as I mentioned, I may become moody, grouchy, hypercritical, and not much fun to be around-maybe, too much lactate or inadequate hydration the previous day or from my last hard work out. Getting plenty of rest, minimising stress, and eating sufficiently is vital. Drinking plenty of water helps wash out lactate, the breakdown product of intensive sometimes anaerobic exercising. Do not rely on thirst. Dark urine suggests you need to hydrate. But do not wait until you are thirsty… then, it may be too late.

A sedentary man requires 2–3 litres of fluid on a warm day. An active man in similar temperatures requires from 5 to 10 litres per day. Urine should remain clear. I have learned that drinking fluids as much as I can before, during, and after exercising – especially for exercising longer distances, keeps me hydrated. Eating easily absorbed foods especially carbohydrates immediately after exercising also helps me avoid a cranky brain.

For prolonged exercise, Dr Leon advises cool beverages of complex sugars and hypotonic electrolytes. Hydration should be simple and affordable. There is plenty of hype touting expensive hydration formulas containing complex carbohydrates. I find flavouring my litre water bottle with a half cup cranberry juice is pleasant, inexpensive, and effective.

A complex carbohydrate sports drink contains 14 Grams of carbohydrate, as a combination of sucrose, glucose, and dextrose per eight ounces. A glass of milk can help the body refuel and reduce muscle damage and improve muscle recovery as well. For longer hikes or even long walks, bring along a quickly digestible, complex carbohydrate in a protein bar or gel form, and not a quick fix like a simple sugar candy bar that can produce an insulin surge and quickly lower your glucose level so important to the brain. Depending on calorie needs and intensity of your workout, an easily digested 180 to 250 calorie energy bar containing six to 20 grams casein, soy, or egg protein can give you an energy boost.

Sports gels (100–120 calories) are simple sugars and contain sucrose and glucose. More about this in the Nutrition chapter. If you are at altitude or have encountered unaccustomed climate change but still want to exercise, give yourself plenty of time to acclimatise to the new altitude, humidity, or temperature. Expect several days to adjust to exercising or competition at higher altitude. An athlete may have a two to three-day grace period before experiencing acute altitude sickness (AMS) that can include headache, fatigue, nausea, dizziness, or unaccustomed weakness.

For those of you contemplating climbing Mount Everest, that's when you must worry about high-altitude cerebral edema (HACE), or high-altitude pulmonary edema (HAPE) –As altitude increases from a comfortable 5,000–6500 ft. to 10,000 ft – 40% are at risk of AMS. Experiencing altitude sickness can be extremely uncomfortable. I can attest to the discomfort I experienced hiking at 14,000 feet in Ecuador's Cajas National Park. Nausea, dizziness, and a headache hit me suddenly and took several days of recovery.

Acclimatising to heat and humidity depends on how much you sweat, and your plasma volume – remember, we are 80% water. Adequate hydration and moderating sweating can maintain circulation. Wear the right clothes – preferably not cotton – but rather wicking fabrics that help sustain a stable core temperature. Monitor your heart rate by checking your pulse every so often. One tipoff dehydration is occurring is discovering you have an unusually rapid heart rate – especially when you wake up – compensating for a low plasma volume from dehydration. A similar discovery can indicate overtraining in an athlete.

The progression from benign to life threatening heat stress can be insidious.

- **Heat cramps** – Serious and painful cramps from loss of water and electrolytes from sweating. Early dehydration is just a 5% weight loss and can produce lethargy, anxiety, or irritability.
- **Heat exhaustion** – Dilated pupils, a weak or rapid pulse, nausea, and vomiting. Temperature rises to 103 degrees.
- **Heat stroke** – Life-threatening when body temperature can be over 106°F. Nervous system dysfunction can include seizures and loss of consciousness.

I remember one of my college professors who was from Ghana coming face to face with a minus 32 degree New Hampshire temperature, commenting, "The thing about the cold is that you can always get warm but, where I come from, when it's hot you can never get cool." For those of us who grew up in the cold and snow belt, playing in a snowbank out back, we experienced near frostbite plenty of times. But it did not seem to bother us.

As we age, circulation to our hands and feet often becomes compromised. We may experience vasoconstriction with narrowing and less compliant peripheral vasculature, and an inability to keep our hands warm. If this is a persistent problem, your doctor can prescribe a calcium channel blockers such as Procardia that can dilate the small arterioles in our extremities, and reduce painful, cold hands or feet. Such systems, I found, less disturbing after I switched from gloves to mittens.

I remember all too well my first wife's displeasure when my daughter, "Gabi", and I returned from a nasty, windy ski in zero temperature with her in a backpack. She had the red mottling to her cheeks of frostnip when fat cells get too cold. Frost nip can change into more serious frostbite which is the crystallisation of water in the fatty tissue leading to freezing of the skin and tissues. I WAS in the doghouse but, fortunately her frostnip resolved

The initial symptom of frostbite is numbness and a white or bluish color to the skin. Swelling and blistering can occur. The hands, feet, and face are most frequently affected. A more serious complication may include developing hypothermia. Risk factors include drinking alcohol, smoking, mental health problems, or prior injuries due to cold exposure and frostbite. The mechanism starts with ice crystals and blood clots in the small blood vessels.

Severity is divided into superficial known as 1st and 2nd degree frostbite or deeper injury called 3rd and 4th degree. Mountaineers are especially at risk with prolonged exposure creating such severe frostbite that they may require amputation of fingers or toes. Frost bite does not hurt during freezing, but thawing can be quite painful. I can attest to this after experiencing this on the tip of my nose and cheeks. But then there was penile frostbite… I know! Never again – wind tights forever.

Enjoy running through winter. But, take care. Out-of-door sport stores have great creams they sell that are barriers to protect your nose, face, neck and cheeks. Watch those body parts, especially if you have had frostbite before. As the temperature drops below freezing, special tapes and a cream called Dermatome can protect your nose and cheeks. Buy a Balaclava or a buff to pull over your nose as the wind-chill factor is factored in. Treat a frozen toe or finger by soaking in cool not warm water. Depending on severity, seek medical care. Best to wear goggles or good protective eye gear in the minus temperatures, especially if the wind picks up, to avoid corneal damage.

Wear breathable, wind-resistant clothing with plenty of flaps and vents to wick sweat away from your body. By doing so, you can keep your core temperature stable and avoid hypothermia. Layer. If you are exercising in arctic conditions or even around freezing, wear wind underwear that have a plastic front to protect your privates. Be warned, hypothermia is not just a severe cold weather event. It can occur on an innocent fall or spring day suddenly cooling, or if it is beginning to rain-particularly dangerous if you are wearing the wrong gear like a cotton shirt. Polypropylene fabrics wick best and protects your core temperature. A cotton shirt is no protection once soaked.

This has happened to me when I was once lost in the woods on a long work-out and had not brought fluids. It was getting dark, my compass was of no use, I was wet and began to shiver, an early danger sign of impending hypothermia. I knew I should be concerned. Fortunately, I found my way out and effectively warmed up. Sometimes, it is better to be a tad on the cool side than drowning in sweat. So, if you are out for several hours, stay dry with clothes that wick. Bring extra water and do not forget an easily stuffed shell for an unexpected weather change especially if you are at altitude or above the tree line.

I have the memory of my 350-mile, month-and-a half long "through" hike on the Superior Hiking Trail traveling north a few miles off Lake Superior along the North Shore from Duluth to Canada. It was mid-May and there were no leaves yet, but plenty of early buds on the maples. My adventure serves to confirm how fickle Lake Superior or any northern weather can be. One day was warm enough for no shirt, shorts, and a quick skinny dip in a tannin-colored icy cold stream.

An hour later the temperature plummeted. The wind shifted to the northeast and began to blow. Then, it began to drizzle and, in short order, started to pour. The rain went horizontal. I realised I was beginning to flirt with hypothermia. I knew – I was wet, cold, and had begun to shiver. Compounding my concern, I accidentally had taken a spur trail to a scenic lookout and had lost the main trail. The trail became steep even for a mountain goat. It was almost vertical with slippery boulders but my only ladder to the top of Carlton Peak.

The Superior Hiking trail has none of the altitudes of The Appalachian or the Pacific Crest National Scenic Trail, but descents and ascents over cascading gorges may be tougher than the White mountains or Cascades. My clothes were ready for the spin cycle. As I reflect how I lived, I came to believe my survival was a Higher Power thing.

The two older folks – I was 72, mind you, approached me wearing two black garbage bag raincoats, their heads popping out from slits. They explained as they passed that I had missed the main trail. Wet, cold, and exhausted – yet, still optimistic – I went my way, and they theirs. Only ten minutes later, I realised my game was over. Nothing on me was dry. There was no dry wood to make a fire. The woods too were drenched. I knew my sleeping bag was beyond wet and useless now.

That is when my two saviours reappeared as if they were giving me another chance. They offered me a ride to dry land. I knew beforehand that there was no way anyone would pick me up on the highway. I was dirty, wet, and cold, and maybe I looked dangerous. Lucky, some folks still pick up hitchhikers– even dirty and wet like I was.

Gone are the days on the farm when the adage that if you must exercise at the end of the day, you have not worked hard enough. We live in a beyond-industrialised, sedentary age of electronic everything. More than ever before, we need to find accessible and effective ways to relieve stress and tension as well as continue, resume, or start anew cardioprotective activity. We must find alternative ways to stay fit and strong.

Serious mood disorders like anxiety, depression, bipolar disorder – the dysphoria's-- can affect how we feel about ourselves, our loved ones, or our co-workers. They can affect how we think. Too much exercise can take its toll too. Exercise mostly affects mood positively or, sometimes, in excess, negatively. Sometimes, too much may not be better. The intensity of how I exercise can negatively affect me. Exercising judiciously generally makes me feel better than if I had slouched for a week on the couch. This notion goes out the window if I overdo it. More likely than not, too long or excessively hard long workouts can take their toll on my mood.

Modern-day tractors, worth many thousands of dollars, have every convenience including air-conditioning, a sound system with boomers and tweeters, and you always have your cell phone at the ready. Farming once lacked such accoutrements.

Farming has gone corporate and big scale as exercise and fitness have declined as numbers of fast food emporiums have escalated. Small farming has become financially borderline. In this noble profession, depression and suicide have escalated. Rural and urban populations must equally participate in convenient and effective exercise. With the current COVID-19 epidemic, farm, city, and suburban couples of every size and color appear to have taken to walking. I notice plenty of couples even holding hands, many with children in tow. Any kind of aerobic and strength workout can serve as an antidote to current emotional, political, financial, or health care instability. Committing to a realistic and safe exercise program can help prevent heart disease, diminish stress, avoid depression and anxiety, or—if you are fortunate—improve relationships.

Statistics in the *Resource Manual for Guidelines for Exercise Testing* offering exercise programming from The College of Sports Medicine (ACSM), are pessimistic even worrisome. They report of dropout rates of 12% from exercise programs in the first three months, and as high as 87% by 12 months. But, I want to remain optimistic that societal attitudes can change.

At the risk of being redundant, helping make a commitment to exercise succeed is to consider a pre-exercise medical assessment and, perhaps, a stress test. If your sports-minded physician recommends a stress test as we are over 60, get one. After All my warnings and enticements, I hope you have decided to exercise. Include enough warm-up and cool-down in your regimen. Stretch before, during, and after your muscles are warmed up. Whatever now motivates you, exercise alone or with others. An exercise specialist, fitness instructor, or coach can design an exercise program that suits your abilities and goals. Start a realistic program so you do not quit. More is not always better. Start low and slow.

In programs such as those provided by The American Lung Association Runners Club, willing volunteers gladly show you how to run and train right so you can complete your first half or full marathon. There are many advantages for entering a local training program: deriving a sense of accomplishment, or just finding a community who will reinforce healthy life changes, such as problems with drinking, smoking, poor sleeping, or bad eating habits.

A Jillian Michaels or a Barre Shred circuit training session at a military-style boot camp before work can be a challenging option. These options combine gut-wrenching aerobics of lung searing jumping jacks, and intense running in place interspersed with push-ups, hand weights, kettle bells that will put you through your strength paces. Alternatively, you can make several circuits around the machines at the gym, or at home do push-ups, pull-ups, or any homespun technique to use your own body for resistance. You can increase aerobic benefits of all such techniques by shortening the time between set or disciplines.

Biking inside on different types of stationary bikes or taking spin classes in this era of dangerous texting while driving, can be safer than risking your life on the road. Take care biking at dusk or on the trail if it is over black ice or loose gravel. Preferably, stay on bike paths. Biking is fine yet can be weather dependent. Mountain and fat tire biking has made the sport safer, extends the season, offering access to challenging terrain season round.

Patience has not been one of my virtues. However, persistence should be your new buzz word how to achieve, renew, or maintain healthy goals. Gradually increase your physical activity over whatever time feels good for you. There is no magic bullet.

Create a fitness program and goal that is realistic. Maybe, it is going to take a month, or maybe, several, even a year progressing up the exercise ladder. I would rather see you start low and slow and continue at it than high and fast and quitting. This is the best way to avoid unnecessary pain and then bailing. One esteemed rheumatologist, marathon runner, and avid ski coach, the late Doctor John Bland, shared with me. "A younger athlete deconditions faster than someone sixty-to-eighty like you and me." Yes, there is a cause for optimism.

If you are hurting and need some rest; do not hesitate to take a break rather than believing that by continuing to exercise or train, you will feel better not worse. A sensible fitness program will work for you. Just look at those youngsters with boundless energy. Those of us over 60 have as much to gain from strength and aerobic training as those kids or anybody in their teens, thirties, or fifties. Just get out there and try it!

Chapter 15
Training Options

– George Sheehan, author, *Running and Being* wrote,
Running is just such a monastery, a retreat, a place to commune with God and
yourself, a place for psychological and spiritual renewal."

– George Sheehan, author of *Running and Being*

So, here we are. We have explored the benefit of several types of training. We have looked at stretching and weight training. *Men Over 60: Don't Quit Now!* has offered safer ways to exercise. Let's say no to "America, we sit". There are plenty of ways to thread the needle toward fitness. I still advise you to always making exercise fun

"Every day running can become the healthiest day of your life," says Dr George Sheehan. There are plenty of ways to thread the needle toward fitness.

My dear friend, Odd Osland, laughs, it is no longer what we said after 9/11, "United we stand," but sadly, "United we sit." We will talk about America's eating habits in the nutrition chapter. Other cultures walk, hike, skate, ski, often as a family. We watch sports rather than doing them. We sit in our folding chairs, thermos of hot coffee in hand – now social distancing-- as we watch our grandchildren playing soccer, baseball, or football.

We have plenty of shrines to athleticism in all the major cities such as the Twin Cities. Locally, hey include the Twin's Target Field, the Saint Paul Saint's CHS Field, the Wild's Excel Energy Stadium, and the Minnesota United FC Allianz Field soccer stadium. There are 762 fitness centres in Minnesota with the sixth-highest number of clubs per capita according to the International Health, Racquet & Sports Club Association. Three Taj Mahal orthopaedic centres cater to a myriad of orthopaedic problems.

As mentioned, Silver and Fit or Silver Sneakers offered free by most supplemental health policies, provide a great opportunity for the over-sixty set to stay fit alone or with like-minded contemporaries. Home exercise equipment is a better investment than term life insurance; that is, if you use them. The once-popular NordicTrack ends up collecting dust as one of the best clothes hangers in the bedroom.

Either at home or at the gym, many exercise machines are a great place to read books or magazines while you are panting away. In the day, cities constructed circuit courses in the parks. Such outdoor playgrounds for adults were a quick and dirty way to work out by using your own weight hanging on bars and beams, or doing push-ups, and pull-ups as you race around the course.

Ken Cooper suggested that we could accomplish aerobic fitness just by exercising 30 minutes a day. Again, start low and slow, and follow Dr. George Sheehan's example how to stay or become aerobically fit and share his love for running.

- Weeks 1–3 – Walk 15 minutes, three times a week.
- Week 4 – Now, jack it up to 20 minutes, three times a week.
- Week 5 – Increase to 25 minutes three times a week (Walk. No need to run or jog yet).
- Week 6 – Now, you are up to that magic 30 minutes a day three times a week. Do not run or jog yet. Walk but you can increase your speed for the same distance.
- Week 7 – Now you are ready to move to jogging; that is, if you felt no shortness of breath, chest discomfort, or significant body pain at the earlier levels. Go for it. Try to decrease the time for your run distances.
- Do not rush it. It may have taken 20 years for you to get out of shape and trying to get back into shape in 20 days can be dangerous or, worse yet, fatal.
- "Beginning runners should start with two to four runs per week at about 20 to 30 minutes (or roughly 2 to 4 miles) per run. You may have heard of the 10% rule—You should never increase your weekly (running) mileage by more than 10% over the previous week-- but a better way to increase your mileage is to do so every second week. This will help your body adapt to your new hobby, so you don't get hurt."
- Love you, Dr. Sheehan. You deserve a special place in heaven for helping so many of us discover that "Every day running is the best day of our lives."

Although swimming is a great aerobic exercise, it is not weight bearing and will not prevent osteoporosis. Swimming is a great break to give your program variety and is not as punishing to your body. The Stairmaster is also a low-impact aerobics step program. However, either has an advantage over a complacency of starting or maintaining fitness.

Do not get hurt. Make it fun. Do it alone or with a group of like-minded men and women, your children, or grandchildren. Do not just watch. Do! Create a perfect program with realistic goals by yourself or with professional assistance for weight loss, stopping smoking, or handling stress. If you are determined to become or remain competitive, there are still advantages by training smart despite passing the sixty milepost. Certainly, if you have the persistence to stay in the competition game, you will have less competition and can take some hardware home. Now, by taking the challenge to stay fit, there can be a guarantee for joy feeling stronger and healthier each day. The competition is now within.

Chapter 16
Nutrition – You Are What You Eat

This chapter describes the best foods to maintain muscle mass, bone integrity, ideal weight, a feeling of fullness, and satiety. Food should look and taste good and still be healthy. Exercise demands attention to and managing hydration. There are healthy and palatable alternatives to the traditional American diet unfortunately, high in saturated fats. Reverse the custom of using vegetables to flavour meat. Try the reverse, let meat flavour your veggies. The need for supplements and extra vitamins and minerals—unnecessary at regular activity levels as an addition to fresh fruits and vegetable, may increase with demanding physical activities, or on vegetarian and vegan diets. Consider alternatives like the Mediterranean diet. Drink in moderation. Don't forget hydration—after all, we are 80% water.

"Primates need good nutrition, to begin with. Not only fruits and plants, but insects as well."
– Richard Leakey, paleoanthropologist, conservationist

We can be overwhelmed by different diet possibilities: the Atkins, Paleo, Mediterranean, Okinawa, Vegan, Vegetarian, and many other options. So, let us quickly review premier diets. Lacto-vegetarians eschew meat but consume milk products and eggs. Pescatarians (not just Presbyterians) also eat fish but eschew other meats. Vegans do not eat any animal products. The tenets of animal veneration by Buddhists are why all those cows are walking peacefully and unafraid around the streets of India. Mr. Roberts was a vegetarian saying he would not eat anything that had a mother. Later he decided that he would not eat anything with eyes. Personally, I will eat any animal that volunteers. I wonder how many carnivores would replace meat with vegetables if they had to slaughter the cow for their next McDonald's Whopper?

I try not to eat my politics but am not always successful at my bid to be apolitical over dinner. Frightened by the similarity between human and animal, I quit eating meat for a year after my rotation in orthopaedic surgery in medical school. Within the past few years, I resumed a vegetarian diet, and have been pleasantly satisfied. Granted, a diet without meat requires some ingenuity combining, cooking, and eating complementary amino acids that comprise the beans and rice combination that has satisfied much of the Third World for centuries. Such a preference is associated with a lower prevalence of heart disease.

There are other environmental reasons for choosing not to eat meat. We are in the era of mega farms. Growing beef, pigs, and chicken expends enormous energy resources, creates animal waste that contaminates and depletes ground water, as well, and with certain animals like cows, produces significant amounts of CO_2. If you want to eat meat or fish, buy free-ranging animals or fish farmed in sustainable environments.

A Mediterranean diet of plant-based foods promoted by University of Minnesota epidemiologists such as K-Ration inventor, Ansel Keyes, and later, Dr Henry Blackburn of the University of Minnesota, offers strategies for heart-healthy living. The Mediterranean Diet has been the basis of a diet rich in fruits, vegetables, complex carbohydrate such as in whole grain breads and cereals, fish, lamb, olive oil, and red wine. Cardioprotective and longevity-associated benefits are patterned after the diet and lifestyle of pastoral Greek shepherds – not someone sitting all day at an office job.

This is a diet low in saturated fats, cholesterol, derived from not-so-lean meat. "The times they are a changing," Bob Dylan tells us. Rates of obesity have risen as abundance in more economically developed countries runs rampant. Meta-analyses of over 1.5 million healthy adults on the Mediterranean diet report a reduced risk of cardiovascular mortality and overall morbidity.

If you decide on a vegetarian or vegan diet, eat vegetables rich in iron such as broccoli, string beans, dark leafy vegetables such as collard greens, kale, and spinach, and tomato paste, among others. Iron in haemoglobin is vital for effective physical performance. Eighty % of iron is effectively absorbed from the small intestine and incorporated into haemoglobin, a protein found in red blood cells, that carries vital oxygen to organs and muscles. The iron comprising "heme" in meat is more effectively absorbed from the bowel than plant iron. Vitamin C, and vitamin A in red peppers, strawberries, orange juice, or watermelon enhance iron absorption.

Iron assists immune function and builds enzymes for DNA synthesis. Haemoglobin is vital for enhancing muscle myoglobin. A man needs 8 milligrams of iron a day. We recirculate red cells that contains iron every 150 days.

"How do vegans and vegetarians get enough iron?'" I asked another knowledgeable physician.

His answer was succinct.

"With great difficulty."

As a fish-consuming vegetarian and long-standing endurance athlete, I have had decades of a borderline low haemoglobin; a low total serum iron, an occasionally low ferritin level – the protein that carries iron, – and a borderline percentage saturation, a quantitative level assuring that the protein that stores iron is adequately filled. Maintaining an acceptable haemoglobin can be compromised by diet or bleeding anywhere in the GI tract. An anaemia, however, in a man over sixty-, unless proven otherwise – by an upper and lower GI series or endoscopy, can be a bowel bleed as from a cancer. In my case, and after a normal colonoscopy, a 325 mg iron tablet once or twice a day has maintained my haemoglobin sufficient to maintain my exercise regimen and excel competitively.

Cereals and flour have been reinforced with iron for a long time. Just a meal of clams or oysters can provide 100% of the required daily iron allowance (RDA). One cup of cooked white beans or lentils, or lightly cooked spinach provides 20% RDA of iron.

The Mayo Clinic has promoted the Dash Diet that includes 27% of total calories as fat, 18% as protein, and 55% as carbohydrate, with plenty of fruits, vegetables, and low-fat dairy products. The Okinawan Diet emphasises soy products, fish, and seaweed. The Japanese have had the lowest cardiovascular disease (CVD) and cancer rates worldwide. Their diet includes plenty of leafy green vegetables, fruits, and green tea. Eastern countries particularly China, have always had lower rates of colon cancer; that is, until McDonalds and saturated fats arrived.

I do not endorse fad weight reduction diets. *Men Over 60:Don't Quit Now!* recommends balancing a healthy diet with exercise. Atkins and other low-carbohydrate-high fat and protein diets like the Keto Diet may keep insulin levels low; yet, like The Atkins Diet can cause ketosis; that is, when the body metabolises fat and protein and not carbohydrates for energy. This diet is not recommended for high-performance athletes. The several days of only a diet of protein and fat, for example, in "carbo loading, can play havoc with an endurance athlete when the brain runs out of glucose before beginning the hyper compensation phase with only glucose, known as "carbo loading.",—that reputedly, can build glycogen stores for the big race ahead.

The "Poor Man's Hamburger" of Peanut butter and honey on two slices of eight-grain bread, has no cholesterol and two grams of fibre. It is cheaper than meat and the discerning shopper can find the spread without corn syrup, preservatives, a simple sugar, or extra oil. Nut protein like peanut butter provides essential amino acids that your body does not produce. You do not get the same calories or saturated fat, the "bad guys", from nuts as from even lean cuts of meat. Nuts are high in monounsaturated fats, the "good guys", as well as providing a great source of protein. Protein from nuts becomes complete when combined with a multigrain bread. Nuts also contain important vitamins and minerals.

The key is to consume a varied diet. A tablespoon of either almond or peanut butter is equivalent to one ounce of protein and equivalent to an ounce of red meat minus the cholesterol. Peanut and almond butter are also rich in vitamin E, an antioxidant, that prevents free radicals from oxidising deoxyribonucleic acid (DNA). Although almonds and peanuts are quite caloric, they are high in dietary fibre. Almonds contain 25.6 mg per 100 grams and peanuts 4.9 per 100 grams of fibre as well as impressive amounts of magnesium that facilitates muscle contractions, enhances bone health, and enhances metabolism.

Unsalted peanuts, walnuts, macadamia nuts, or almonds, are packed with heart-healthy monosaturated fats – omega-3-fatty acids, alpha linoleic acid, proteins, vitamins, and minerals with 160 calories/ounce – 23 nuts have 5 grams of protein. Brazil nuts provide 100% of the daily requirement of an essential micronutrient and powerful antioxidant, selenium. A 2006 study suggests that walnuts are as effective as olive oil at reducing inflammation and oxidation in arteries. A new twist. "A walnut a day, keeps the myocardial infarction away."

I have fish one or two meals a week. I poach, carefully broil, bake, but never fry or barbecue my fish that produce free radicals that can be carcinogenic. Our taste buds love fried food – battered and deep-fried anything. Drop by the fast-food drive-in of your choice for your daily fix for all the above. Many fast-food chains now list a calorie content for their foods. I am an unabashed food snob. I am as vigilant as possible of what I put into my body. I am still a sucker though for ice cream. I seem to need the calories to maintain my weight. Exercising hard and eschewing meat gives me some slack.

Sarcopenia is the loss of muscle with age. Diet can be a vital prevention. Recommended daily allowance (RDA) of muscle-building protein is 0.8 g/kg per day amounting to 56 grams/day for a 70kg man. The number jumps for an endurance athlete to 1.2–1.3 g/kg/day, at least for the first 2–4 weeks of training, and to 1.5–2g/kg/day for intense strength training.

Grains combined with complimentary amino acids as in legumes, have been the world's source of protein for 40,000 years. For vegans and vegetarians, the question arises, do we have enough protein in our diets to build muscle.? Vegans eating a varied diet of vegetables, beans, grains, nuts, and seeds rarely have any difficulty getting enough protein if their diet contains enough energy calories to maintain weight. Admittedly, such a diet requires careful planning to incorporate essentials such as Vitamin B12 and iron. If you are vegetarian, you may need to beef up your eating to feel full, if you excuse the reference to the more typical US diet.

You do not need to eat foods containing complimentary amino acids at one sitting but should do so over the ensuing 24 hours. Try to eat a varied diet. Regretfully, non-meat sources of protein for the average American provide as little as 16–20% of the daily diet. Americans flavour their meat with vegetables while Eastern cultures flavour their vegetables with meat. A reality bite is that eating red meat has an increased risk of developing colon cancer, type 2 diabetes, and coronary heart disease.

Legumes, nuts, and seeds contain about 20–30 grams of protein per one-cup serving. A cup of 85% lean beef has 22 grams of protein. Most of the soybean crop stretching as far as the eye can see in any midwestern field will head to the Far East. Soy products such as tofu, tempeh, or soy burgers, for instance, are easily digestible, low in saturated fats, and provide adequate protein.

Exciting food science has produced a palatable and deceptively scrumptious plant-based "meat" alternative to beef. Among the players, Beyond Beef, Morning Star Farms' Incogmeato, Impossible Burger, and Beyond Meat are the rising culinary stars. The manufacturers of the plant-based Impossible Burger attribute its flavour and hue to soy leghaemoglobin, a protein made from genetically modifying yeast. It even appears to bleed, and is now available at many chains including Burger King, now home of the "Impossible Whopper". Currently, plant-based meat can cost twice as much as lean beef.

Plant-based alternatives are still pretty spendy. Retail sales of meat alternatives in the U.S were $4.5 billion as of July, 2019, and are predicted to grow to $85 billion by 1930. Companies like Cargill and Tyson are scooping up start-ups of the alternative meat developers. They are taking off running in the sustainable alternative "meat" industry.

A word of caution is due about the new plant-based "meat". One purveyor, Beyond Meat's 4-ounce patio, is 270 calories. A similar weight lean beef equivalent weighs in at 280 calories. Protein is the same for "meat, containing more fibre. However, the plant-based burger is higher in sodium than a hamburger. They have equal amounts of saturated fat. Pound-for-pound, alternative meat is more expensive.

Just hit the shelves at your grocery store and see cases and cases of meat, less expensive than the plant-based alternatives, and equally simple to prepare. Animal meat is a complete protein, so you do not have to combine the 9 essential amino acids as you must with rice and beans. The negative impact-- an environmental footprint of animal waste, water diversion, diversion of soy and corn as feed for animals not people, is the result of massive cattle, hog, and chicken corporate operations that are non-sustainable, and also play a part in further polluting our environment. Here I go again, eating my politics.

The bottom line is that plant-based meats are more processed, more expensive, and significantly higher in sodium (370 mg for the Impossible Burger) than a lean beef patty (72 mg). A beef patty and a Beyond Burger in particular, are tied at 6g saturated fat. Nutritionally, ethically, environmentally, if you want an honest health food fix, go for the original black bean patty or bean burger that are less processed and are not made with the highly saturated fat like coconut oil

The downside is that a meat alternative like veggie soy burgers, soy hotdogs, marinated tofu, or tempeh kabobs with fruit or veggies, may not provide the same olfactory arousal as a "Juicy Loosie". Yet, soy alternatives work well either plain or flash-seared with rice as a stir fry. Mock duck or fry-hardened firm tofu are readily available and, if presented creatively, are healthy and enjoyable meat substitutes. I /must confess that the aromatic smell of charring beef smoke from my neighbour's barbecue can be as enticing for me as were the Sirens, Scylla and Charybdis, and the Cattle of the Sun, to Odysseus.

I encourage combining grains and legumes but careful to include dairy or eggs high in protein, iron, and vitamin B12. If you choose to be vegan, it is circumspect to take supplements. Phenylalanine, valine, threonine, tryptophan, methionine, leucine, isoleucine, lysine, and histidine are the essential amino acids we do not synthesise and must be present in our food to combine with nonessential amino acids to make proteins.

The essential trace element, selenium is high in Brazil nuts, fish, milk products, eggs, and the universal food du jour, brown rice, and beans. If in doubt, stressed, or on a pure vegan diet, there is value in taking a reputable multivitamin supplement containing iron, iodine, fluoride, copper, zinc, chromium, selenium, manganese, and molybdenum.

The classic food pyramid has been replaced by MyPlate (www.dietaryguidelines.gov).MyPlate by the U.S. Government Departments of Agriculture and Health and Human Services (USDA and USDHHS) as Guidelines for Selection of a Nutritionally-Sound Health-Promoting diet. The plan is divided into 5 sections: vegetables, fruits, grains, protein, and dairy. The diet suggests two-thirds plant products – whole grains, fruits, vegetables and one-third animal protein sources.

MyPlate advises limiting fat intake to 25–35% of the overall diet and avoiding fats that harden at room temperature – especially trans fats. Twenty to 35% of your daily calories should be protein. Go lean and mean. Take a pass on the fatty meat. Instead, eat leaner turkey-based bacon and sausage. Twenty-five % of calories should be carbohydrate from the grain family but, of a dense variety that includes choices like eight-grain bread, whole wheat noodles, and brown rice.

Eat foods high in fibre. Avoid simple sugars and short-chain carbohydrates like white flour that can increase the risk for metabolic problems such as diabetes. Count your calories. Nutritionists advise that men eat 2,400 to 3,000 calories a day and women 1,800 to 2,200 calories a day.

The U.S. tops calorie intake compared with the rest of the world, averaging 3,770 calories a day. All too many advertisements crowd the airways with enticing ads for ubiquitous comfort foods like crispy fried chicken dipped in creamy something or other, or a myriad of unhealthy choice like a build-your-own "Supreme" cheese-packed pizza. All are cleverly designed to press your yummy food button. We are not dying from starvation but from abundance. Certain groups such as Hmong immigrants, once an agrarian mountain culture, now quantify their success and wealth by how much meat, usually pork, they consume.

My doctors had warning signs from my total cholesterol levels over several decades-- repeatedly over 200mg% (Normal 125–200mg%). None prescribed a statin or suggested modifying my diet. No one who had treated me over those decades, reacted to my total cholesterol and worrisome elevated low-density lipoprotein (LDL)– despite continuing exercise and maintaining ideal weight combined with an acceptable high-density lipoprotein (HDL) level over 40mg% (the "good" cholesterol), prescribed a statin.

My rude awakening was sudden angina on an easy walk with my wife. An angiogram showed that both the left anterior descending coronary artery ("The Widow Maker"), and the circumflex artery, which both supply the hefty left ventricle were blocked. My cardiologist immediately inserted two stents into the offending arteries. All this seemed counter-intuitive. I considered myself a committed and well-trained athlete. The answer was a resounding yes. However, this had become a time of huge personal, financial, and professional stress for me. Let us call this a graphic example of the mind-body connection.

In addition to several losses and setbacks, my lipid abnormalities had caught up with me. As do many with elevated total cholesterol and LDL, I had an all-too-common genetic deficiency, familial hypercholesterolemia, a defect on

170

chromosome 19, that makes the body unable to remove low density lipoprotein (LDL) cholesterol. For the most part, the problem had less to do with my diet and more to do with heredity. Perhaps, the calcified plaques could have been prevented with more aggressive measures: a low cholesterol diet or, if indicated, as in my case, a statin.

What happened to me at that stage of my life were shots over the bow to my chemistry, and influenced to a certain extent, by my lifestyle and circumstances at the time. Blood cholesterol can be influenced by genetics, weight, age, smoking, physical activity, or eating habits. I have been symptom free since the stents and taking a statin. Twenty years later, each ski marathon I complete is another confirmatory stress test.

Statins such as Lipitor (atorvastin), Lescol (fluvastin), Pravachol (pravastin). My yearly total cholesterol and LDH (calculated) level this year on atorvastin are now 165 and 93 mg/dl, respectively, with no further heart complications. However, some physicians would advise a LDL lower than 70mg % and a baby aspirin daily.

Eat foods high in nutrient density (ND), and choose from among nutrient-dense fat-free fruits, dark green, red, and orange veggies such as squash, kale, chard, spinach, leafy greens combined with whole grains, low-fat dairy, nuts and seeds, lean meat, or legumes combined with complex carbohydrates like beans and brown rice, the latter to produce a complete protein. Do not forget onions that are shock full of sulphides as ideal phytochemicals producing cancer-fighting antioxidants.

Choose a multigrain sandwich roll at Subway instead of a processed low nutrient dense bread made from white flour. Ask for brown rice at your favourite Indian or Chinese restaurant (lots of luck on that one) rather than white race that has had all its nutrients ripped off. MyPlate recommends healthy body weight by limiting the volume, and composition of food. Consult the charts for that.

Nutritionists advise drinking 1% milk. Try cultured milk in the form of kefir and avoid highly caloric sugary beverages.

Alcohol, to drink or not to drink? The late Jay Phillips, scion of the Phillips Beverage Company, attached to his bottles "Drink in moderation." Depending on your weight, gender, and race, a man, can drink one to two glasses of wine or beer a day. If you are French, the deal is off. Do not be fooled. An ounce of distilled liquor has the same alcohol content as a glass of wine or a bottle of beer. I recommend zero tolerance which means not drinking if you plan to drive. Your bartender is not your best friend when he gives you a double shot because he "likes" you. You or one of your friends could have a drinking problem if it leads to problems in a relationship, in school, in social activities, or how you think or feel. Remember, alcohol, especially in excess, is a depressant.

Life is all too short. Eat reasonable portions, avoid saturated fats, and EXERCISE regularly. But I think I may have said that before. Go with the whole grains. Make it whole wheat. Try a whole wheat Everything Bagel with low-fat cream cheese or, perhaps, feta. Eat peanut or almond butter unadulterated with unnecessary corn syrup or stabilisers.

Reading labels and checking the composition of the food you plan to eat should be your mantra. Gluten intolerance has become the 21st century's epidemic, or is it a fad? There are other explanations for a "bread belly". Maybe, too much beer? Maybe, too much fat; that is, comfort food. The true epidemic is excessive weight and a lack of fitness beginning as adolescents, or even earlier, and continuing into our 60s.

Enjoy your meal or a special treat but, eat with care. As our ancestors who fought the wholly mammoths had to survive, eat to live rather than living to eat. This has become a tall order in a sedentary culture of overabundance.

I look at the long queue of cars lined up for breakfast, lunch, or dinner at fast food drive-up windows, especially during the epidemic. I understand that tired, working parents know that comfort foods will make their kids content regardless of the health consequences. I hope this chapter will assist in your food choices, pleasure, and ultimate better health.

Exercise accompanied by satisfying healthy food can make you feel better and, hopefully, achieve better health. Make your exercise fun and your diet enticing. Just make the best choices you can. If you suspect your diet is not helping you achieve a healthy weight, have your physician refer you to a competent nutritionist. Such a referral can be included in your health plan. Just ask. Good food, pleasant exercise, and, let us not forget, satisfying sex release naturally occurring feel-good endorphins that will enhance your mood and sense of well-being. As is said in Yiddish by a nurturing Jewish mother, "Zi gazunt, .Enjoy!"

Chapter 17
Medical Illnesses of Men Over 60

Don't fear irreversible medical changes. Exercise lowers blood pressure, coronary artery disease, strokes, and heart attacks. Do your best to achieve optimal weight. Watch your cholesterol. Get a colonoscopy every 10 years starting at 50. React to continuing body changes. Heart disease kills more men over 60 than cancer, stroke, chronic lung disease, accidents, infections, diabetes, suicide, kidney disease, or chronic liver disease. Moving into our sixties, you should expect an EKG and, if at risk, a cardiac stress test at your next physical. Current evidence-based drug protocols have revolutionised cancer treatment. Achieve bone health. STDs do happen in men over 60. Periodontal disease, addiction, and skin cancer have consequences regardless of age or socioeconomic status.

"Old Age and sickness bring out the essential characteristics of a man."
– Felix Frankfurter, Associate Justice, The Supreme Court (1939–1962)

In *Men Over 60: Don't Quit Now!* we began with a man's fear of dying. I am speaking from a doctor's perspective akin to "The man who knew too much". Every odd twitch, momentary pain, or compromising skin blotch often provokes in me a knee jerk that can be amplified into a fatal premonition of a hopeless outcome, and a temptation to call my doctor at two in the morning. Instead, I surf the internet for a more realistic explanation. Usually, I return to my happy place once I confirm I do not have such an imagined and often esoteric terminal illness. Yet, as soon as I take a big bite of reality, relieved, I move on with my life.

Generalities About Worrying

Why should men over 60 worry more than our younger counterparts? "Why am I short of breath?" "Why does my back hurt when I wake up?" "How come half the orchestra is darker than the other?" (As when I discovered I had cataracts) during a requiem at Orchestra Hall. "Why does everyone need to repeat what they just told me... but louder?" Compartmentalise worrisome physical changes:

- **Awareness** and **acceptance** of real changes to our bodies or our minds that accompany normal ageing, and that we must live with. Let us call these the realities of ageing.

- **Reversible** – These are concerns that, if we adhere to heathy behaviours, the outcome can be changed for the better. *Men Over 60: Don't Quit Now!* explains to a man past 60 how healthy living can enhance our lives. We need to go face-on with misconceptions about how capable we are and, with directed effort, that we will not lose the big fight. We may need to educate our physician and others, who erroneously believe age-related stereotypes that we lack the goods to thrive with the sunset peeking over the horizon. After we have solicited a clean bill of health, begin, renew, and maintain an exercising commitment. Self-renewal is attainable. This chapter endeavours to reach any man over 60, and is intended to be relevant and understandable. If you stay fit, achieve optimal weight, keep an eye on your cholesterol level, you are more likely to live unscathed well over 60 and, of we are optimistic, into our 90s. I am specifically speaking to men concerned about their health, who want to understand techniques and scientific advances that may reverse what is medically correctable in their lives.

Heart Disease

Heart disease is the leading cause of death among those of us over 60. It supersedes cancer, stroke, chronic lung disease, accidents, infections, diabetes, suicide, kidney disease, and chronic liver disease.

The American Heart Association (AHA) includes high blood pressure in the definition of heart disease. The prevalence of hypertension among men 85 to 90 is 80%, and represent a major risk factor for strokes and heart attacks. Fortunately, it is one of those challenges that may be ameliorated. The mortality gap between women and men has been steadily diminishing. Now, heart disease is the leading cause of death in women over 65(21.9% versus 20.3% from cancer among non-Hispanic women). Since 1984 more women have died from heart disease than men. Women tend to outlive men, distorting the statistics.

Lifestyle changes can correct hypertension. Exercise lowers blood pressure. Family history is a major risk factor. Review your family tree for heart disease. The message is that we need to identify our family history Continue to check your lipids. Exercising and diet increases HDL and helps lower total cholesterol and LDL. Worry less and do more by correcting elevated lipids, losing weight, exercising, quitting smoking and, if necessary, begin cholesterol-lowering medications. We can do a great deal to decrease risk factors for coronary artery disease and by doing so, correct what we can. Why not? worry less!

High blood pressure affects one of three adults in the U.S. The American College of Cardiology considers 120/90 the blood pressure that will reduce the risk of stroke, heart failure, and all-cause mortality. Your healthcare provider pays more attention now, to your systolic blood pressure rather than your diastolic, the lower blood pressure. On a chance visit to the clinic, your blood pressure may be above these limits. There is no reason to panic. Some people just become frightened, called "white coat" hypertension. Get it retested at your pharmacy or the fire house. Owning your own blood pressure cuff can conveniently monitor this controllable life changer.

The National Heart, Lung, and Blood Institute suggests ways to lower blood pressure. Here's what to do for starters to allay avoidable fears. Consult tables and aim for an ideal weight and body mass index relating to your height and weight. Limit salt in your diet. Try the Mayo DASH Diet (Dietary Approaches to Stop Hypertension) that is rich in vegetables, fruits, and other plant-based, unprocessed foods and containing 2400 mg salt a day. The next advisement can be a tough one for a three-cup a day "Joe" lover; that is to limit how much coffee you drink a day, or at least make your second or third cup 50/50, a "half caf." Stop smoking. Follow the one to two drink-a-day rule.

What happens when lifestyle changes such as better nutrition or stress modifications do not control an elevated blood pressure? A doctor often prescribes a diuretic, a water pill, long a frontline medication for hypertension. Should your blood pressure prove refractory, the next tier includes an ACE inhibitors, a beta blocker, calcium channel blockers, vasodilators, alpha blockers, alpha-2 receptor agonists, and central agonists as essential to avoid incipient heart failure or stroke. Ask for supporting and especially evidence-based research about your new antihypertensive. Don't believe television drug commercials. If prescribed, ask your pharmacist about negative interactions with your other drugs. That is, if you can talk to a pharmacist. When it comes to medications, my pharmacist is my best friend. They are ALSO doctors now.

Dr D's Handbook for Men Over 40, described unusual causes for heart failure or a sometimes fatal arrhythmia. An asymptomatic, anomalous coronary artery inadequately supplying blood to the left ventricle, can cause sudden death Congestive Heart Failure in a man at any age. Sudden death in any man can occur during increased physical activity if the left coronary, especially, becomes blocked by plaques. Another reason to attack elevated LDL total cholesterol early and the increasing prevalence of obesity in our society, is to avoid producing plaques and blockage of coronary arteries. Lipid screening is vital for men of all ages, even adolescents and deserves dietary alterations or medication

NBA Hall of Famer, "Pistol Pete" Maravich, collapsed and died while playing pick-up basketball. He died young because he did not have a predominant left coronary artery supplying blood to his left ventricle. In *Dr D's Handbook for Men Over 40,* I identified that a sudden arrhythmia with or without a congenital irregularity of the coronary arteries or ventricular septal dysfunction can cause sudden death of a man in his 40s or younger. Cholesterol-related plaques are of significant concern for men over 60.

Because of reduced physical activity and poor diet, men over 60 may begin developing coronary artery disease earlier. This is a genuine problem that should be addressed as early as possible. Over 60 is not the best time to give up healthy activities, eating right, and achieving ideal weight. Start earlier! We cannot correct the age factor. As ageing men, we are at a greater risk of developing coronary artery disease. This problem is correctible, for example, by stopping smoking – another preventable risk factor. There is a side benefit of stopping smoking, a significant risk factor for heart disease is that after 10 years the risk of lung cancer is the same as for someone who has never smoked. Whew! Fortunately, I stopped smoking at 37. A reality bite is that 37 seems a long time ago.

Men over 60 learn they must accommodate to changes affecting how hard and fast their heart pumps. Although cardiac output at rest is unaffected by age, maximal heart rate declines and is calculated as 220 minus age. Cardiac output, the volume of blood pumped out of the left ventricle is the multiple of stroke volume (the quantity of blood pumped out of the left ventricle with every heart beat) and heart rate. Past 60, a decrease in heart rate affects performance. The ability to increase higher activity levels declines as the volume of blood pumped per minute decreases. As our maximal heart rate declines, we can no longer keep up with the younger pack. We lose speed but, with sufficient training, we can sustain greater endurance capacity. Despite chronic medical problems such as chronic obstructive pulmonary disease, atrial fibrillation, or heart failure, we can still exercise safely.

Men over 60 who chose to compete at the masters level may no longer wish to subject themselves to the pain of gruelling workouts due to the fear of dying, laziness, depression, or accepting cultural misconceptions that we just are too old to do so.

If you have cardiac risk factors and are about to begin a vigorous exercise program or have symptoms of angina, schedule a visit to your physician for an EKG that can show old, recent, or ongoing cardiac muscle injury. If any of these findings appear, your doctor will order a graduated cardiac stress test either on a treadmill or on a recumbent bike. If you are unable to run or bike, medications can increase your heart for the test. Angina can accompany exercise of any intensity, or even from emotional stressors. Someone with an evolving heart attack reports feeling a huge weight on their chest often described as if an elephant were sitting on their chest. Angina is evanescent, coming and going, but premonitory for a myocardial infarction.

A negative ECG stress test can lessen your fear for your safety at your next pick-up hockey game with the guys. Although a negative stress test has no guarantees, it does elevate your heart rate to 85% of your maximum heart rate and is quite safe and diagnostic. You are continuously monitored by a trained technician ready to stop the test if you develop anginal symptoms, unexpected irregular beats, or a sudden drop in blood pressure.

Your physician also watches when the stress test finishes when your heart is recovering, looking for changes that could suggest inadequate blood supply to heart muscle from insufficiently perfused coronaries. The cardiologist may next order a stress echo, a test that detects decreased blood flow from coronary narrowing and how effectively your heart is pumping blood.

Alternatively, you may have a thallium stress test in which radioactive dye measure blood flow and can detect damaged heart muscle. If suspicious, the next step is cardiac catheterisation, which is the gold standard and most accurate test for detecting blockage of your coronary arteries or muscle damage. A relatively new technique, magnetic resonance coronary angiography, is cost saving and less invasive but is less sensitive than an angiogram. It is a helpful screening tool.

Many endurance athletes, after large numbers of endurance races, may develop enlarged, athletic hearts. A heart rate of sixty or lower is called bradycardia, a slow heart rate. It is not unusual for an athlete who may have completed scores of endurance events to have a pulse into the 30s as I do A slow heartbeat in an athlete demonstrates a hefty heart muscle pumping a large amount of blood at a slower rate.

More and more long-distance athletes are developing a fast, irregular rhythm called atrial fibrillation accompanied by increasing shortness of breath while exercising. Such a heart change can spell the end of a racing career with lower endurance capacity. An endurance athlete's heart muscle also sustains recurrent damage to smaller muscle fibres ultimately replacing them with less pliant tissue. The heart may then lose elasticity and pump blood less efficiently. Heart valves can also fail either from earlier injury or infection. subsequently, sending insufficient amounts of blood and oxygen to vital organs.

Metabolic Syndrome (Syndrome X)

Metabolic Syndrome includes the combination of high blood pressure, high blood sugar, increased central obesity ("Dunlaps" disease, again), and abnormal lipids. This is a treatable condition contributing to fatty build-up and plaques in the main coronary arteries. This condition affects 23% of all adults, increasing the risk of heart attacks, diabetes, and stroke. What to do? Syndrome X is one of those medical challenges for men over 60 that can be corrected! Correct your blood sugar and blood pressure with diet and exercise. If necessary, treat an elevated cholesterol with weight loss, exercise, or, if necessary, medications.

Twenty-nine % of men over 60 have hereditary maturity onset (type 2) diabetes, and, as with type 1 juvenile diabetes (insulin dependent), both types of diabetes pose a greater risk for heart disease, stroke, kidney disease, blindness, peripheral nerve, and circulatory problems. The most common symptoms for someone with pre-diabetes – early maturity-onset diabetes - can be feeling tired, becoming increasingly thirsty, and increasing frequency of urination. Type 2 diabetes often can be treated by lifestyle changes such as losing weight accompanied by diet modifications, and exercise. If conservative measures fail, an oral antidiabetic medication such as non-long-acting metformin with or without a sulfonylurea, can increase the sensitivity of muscle cells to insulin and the metabolism of glucose.

Low blood sugar can explain mysterious feelings that include dizziness, and headaches. Hypoglycaemia is often caused by blasts of insulin responding too simple sugars like glucose and may be associated with later diabetes. Such a physical response may also occur from too much prescribed insulin.

The Prostate: Why Do I Have to Get Up Twice a night to pee at Night

Another ageing-related condition is an enlarged prostate, called benign prostatic hypertrophy (BPH). Over 60, most men start developing an enlarging prostate. I suspect mine is the size of a guava melon. Do you have tell-tale symptoms such as frequency, especially at night, urgency, or incomplete emptying after urination? At your yearly physical or sooner, request a digital exam, and if you have these symptoms, your physician may well order an in-office ultrasound of your bladder or send you to a urologist to further determine if you have an enlarged bladder from an obstructing, enlarged prostate. A first approach may be limiting the number of cups of coffee or other liquids (beer or wine are diuretics) with or after dinner

The Prostate-Specific antigen (PSA) is the best test for benign prostate hypertrophy (BPH), inflammation, or cancer, and deciding the value of getting a PSA can be a challenging issue for those of us over 70. The incidence of prostate cancer among men 60 to 79 is 16.7% or one in six men. Getting a prostatic specific antigen (PSA) is age dependent. Testing is advised by age 50 or earlier if you are African American or have a family history of prostate cancer. The United States Preventive Services Task Force (USPSTF) advises —based on life expectancy— that a PSA test is optional over 70.

Options for a man with BPH include a urinary flow test, a postvoid residual volume test determined by an ultrasound of the bladder, or a post void catheterisation to determine how much urine is left in your bladder after voiding. I'll opt for the former. If you've been unable to void, a urodynamic and pressure flow study makes sense—no catheter, please. A cystoscopy to examine the inside of the bladder may be indicated if a urinalysis shows hidden or visible blood (haematuria). Be forewarned that many of these studies must travel through your penis and are moderately uncomfortable. Your urologist will use numbing jelly to minimize any discomfort, or should the cystoscopy be more invasive, conscious sedation as an outpatient is used.

Medications are the first line of attack for symptomatic BPH. Options include initially trying an alpha blocker like Flomax (temulosin) that relaxes muscles in the prostate and bladder. Other medications like 5-alpha reductase inhibitors like Proscar or Propecia (finasteride), block prostate enlarging hormones. If you are bothered by symptoms of BPH, avoid a myriad of drugs with anticholinergic properties like diphenhydramine (Benadryl), an antihistamine, a tricyclic antidepressants, or antipsychotics like chlorpromazine that can shut off the spigot. Here's another chance to ask your pharmacist if a new prescribed is safe if you have frequency.

Recently, it seems that many men I know over 60 have symptoms of frequency, urgency, dribbling, or – more frightening – just can't pee. I recently was unable to urinate shortly after getting home from a minor surgical procedure in which I had conscious sedation and, in a moment of panic by the anaesthesiologist, got a medication to bring up my pulse. As a gonzo endurance athlete, my resting pulse can drop into the mid-30s. That just plain scares the hell out of an anaesthesiologist in the operating room. Minutes after returning home, I just could not pee and was in incredible pain. A neighbour hustled me to the ER. After an excruciating wait, FINALLY They tried to thread a flexible catheter in but they quickly opted for what felt like a roto rooter past my enlarged prostate and opened up my outlet obstruction. I conclude that my pain and discomfort before and after the catheter, could replace water boarding to inspire a confession.

There are some innovative urological procedures that can reverse symptoms of an enlarged prostate or, worse yet, outlet obstruction. These include the prostatic urethral lift procedure (UroLift) that compresses the sides of the prostate away from the urethra. It can be performed in the urologist's office and is touted not to produce erectile dysfunction. Another, perhaps, more appealing procedure, Rezum, Water Vapor Therapy, as well as another technique that includes microwave, laser ablation or enucleative procedures. In the past a transurethral prostatectomy (TURP) was usually the mainstay for treating obstructive BPH or cancer of the prostate. Now, robotics cause the least damage.

Four out of five cases of prostate cancer are detected in an early stage in which the cancer has not spread outside the prostate. Miraculously, the five-year survival for early diagnosed prostate cancer is 100% and detectable with a simple digital exam, a random urinalysis to rule out infection, or an increased PSA, to rule out cancer.

Options for treatment of cancer range from a surgical prostatectomy, radiation-- especially in a man over 70 – or simply observation. Later stages of prostate cancer spread to the spine, the ureters, or the bladder. Other options for treating prostate cancer are hormone therapy, chemotherapy, immunotherapy, or radiation. The caveat worth heeding is that most men die WITH not FROM prostate cancer.

False positive results of an elevated PSA in a man over 70 have implicit danger of a prostate biopsy or prostatectomy that may contribute to post-operative incontinence or erectile dysfunction. Yes, plenty of men have sex after 70. That is why I no longer get a PSA with my yearly preventive health visit.

How Your Lungs Work

In the late 1800s Sir William Osler, the "Godfather" of modern medicine, declared, "Pneumonia is the friend of the old man." Chronic respiratory tract disease is the third leading cause of death for men over 65. This segment of the population will increase from 35 million in 2000 to 71 million in 2030. Respiratory disease including chronic obstructive pulmonary disease(COPD), will also proportionally increase.

COPD, includes refractory asthma, emphysema, and chronic bronchitis. Breathing takes muscle strength, and respiratory muscles age with us. Our lungs become weaker and clear mucous less efficiently. Advanced COPD usually from smoking, leads to dangerously low oxygen levels, frequent lung infections, and heart failure. Chronic asthma may worsen with age. However, all that wheezes is not always asthma. As the heart begins to fail, fluid may collect in the lungs, and, like asthma, produces wheezing and shortness of breath. Treatment of congestive heart failure is different and requires medications to remove fluid from the lungs by strengthening the heart.

Sixty percent of the 24 million with asthma have allergies to pollutants, dust, pollen, exercising in the cold, or from emotional stressors. Acute untreated asthma can kill. An acute burst of a nebulized short-acting beta-agonist like Proventil (albuteral) is called a rescue inhaler as it is an effective bronchodilator. Ed: PP:

Atrovent (ipratropium), an anticholinergic, works for chronic asthma but, if breathing fails to improve, a physician may prescribe a steroid inhaler, prednisone orally or, in acute situations, prednisone intravenously.

Chronic asthmatics benefit from a long-acting inhalable steroid such as fluticasone (Flovent), a long-acting beta agonist such as salmeterol (Serevent), a combination inhaler such as Advair (fluticasone and salmeterol); or,– If the asthma is an allergic variety, – a long-acting leukotriene modifier, Singular (montelukast) can be effective.

Cigarette smoking is linked to about 80–90% of lung cancers. Other tobacco products such as snuff or pipes, increase the risk of mouth and throat cancers. Smokers have a 15–30 times greater chance of developing lung cancer and dying than non-smokers. Repeat: if you haven't smoked for over 10 years, your chances of getting lung cancer approximate those who never smoked. So, if you do smoke, quit!

Ed PP:

Radon, the second leading cause of lung cancer after cigarette smoking, is a naturally occurring radioactive gas responsible for about 21,000 lung cancer-related deaths yearly. You can purchase an inexpensive radon test kit for your home. If radon is detected, you should seek professional advice.

A Brief Overview of Lung Cancers

Listen to your body and act. Oncologists provide successful and evidence-based drug protocols to put you into remission, and, hopefully, a cure. Cancer rates have dropped. Unexplained weight loss, a persistent cough, coughing up blood, shortness of breath, unexplained chest pain, loss of appetite, or unexplained fatigue, are serious issues and if you have any of these signs or symptoms, expect your health professional to schedule an exam including a chest X ray, a complete blood count (CBC), and a chemistry profile.

Non-small Cell Lung Cancer (NSCLC) is the most common lung cancer, representing 85% of all cancers, and has a 5-year survival rate of 92%. Multiple options are available for treatment. Other non-small carcinomas are peripheral adenocarcinoma, squamous cell in the main stem bronchus, and the rapidly growing large-cell undifferentiated carcinoma.

Small cell cancer, also called oat cell, originates in the bronchus, is more prevalent in men over 60, metastasises rapidly, is related to smoking, but can be more responsive to chemotherapy than the other forms of lung cancer. Recently, immunotherapy boosting the body's immune system, has proven to be of value in chemotherapy failures. However, advanced small cell cancer has only an 8% survival rate.

On a less optimistic note, under these and other cancer or other serious medical occurring circumstances for a man over 60, preparing a final directive is always a realistic decision. By doing so, you can make advance decisions in the event of an untreatable condition as to how aggressive you wish your loved ones to be about intubation or resuscitation.

I sadly recall a Dartmouth classmate who attended our 50th reunion knowing he had terminal cancer. This was his farewell to his friends of half a century past. We learned that after his return home he courageously took final comfort medications he and his care team had assembled so he could end his life with dignity.

My father, a lifelong heavy cigarette smoker, developed escalating shortness of breath, and bloody fluid in both lungs that meant he had inoperable metastatic lung cancer. The night after my final visit, he pulled his breathing tube out, developed a respiratory arrest, and died. We believe that my father, a paraplegic from polio and esteemed hospital administrator who had been confined to a wheelchair since his 30s, decided he had enough.

Colorectal Cancer (CRC)

After lung cancer, colon cancer is the second biggest killer of men over 60, with over 200,000 cases per year. Forty thousand men die yearly from colorectal cancer – most between the ages of 65 and 74.

65percent of asymptomatic colorectal cancers can be detected by a simple digital exam at your yearly physical. Also, a haemoglobin below 12.4 gm/dL in a middle-age or older man – especially of the iron-deficient variety – can indicate colorectal cancer, bleeding polyps, or colitis, and warrants both a lower and upper endoscopy. An older man who discovers pencil-thin stools or a change in bowel habit, blood on toilet tissue (not from haemorrhoids), unintended weight loss, or persistent abdominal pain, should consult with a physician. The American Cancer Society recommends a colonoscopy starting at age 45 and then every 10 years, or more frequently if a man has a history of polyps, is African American, or has a family history of colon cancer.

Further colonoscopy beyond age 76 is an individual decision based on health status. Cologuard or FIT immunochemical tests are easier but have more false positives still making colonoscopy still the gold standard.

Other Gastrointestinal Concerns

- Acid reflux and gastritis with heartburn or vomiting can, after an appropriate work-up, be treated with over-the-counter medications such as antacids, proton pump inhibitors like omeprazole, or an H2 blocker like ranitidine that can reduce stomach acid and are available at reduced strength over the counter

Peptic ulcers and cancer – The average age of developing stomach cancer is 68. We can anticipate that 27,510 cases of stomach cancer will be diagnosed annually in men over 65. A parasite, Helicobacter pylorus (H pylori), is strongly linked to gastritis, ulcers, and stomach cancer as are smoking and obesity Antioxidants such as vitamin C, beta carotene, vitamin E, and the mineral, selenium, remove dangerous free radicals associated with cancers. Replacing heavily salted or smoked meats high in nitrites, and eating plentiful fresh fruits and vegetables have lessened the risk of gastric cancer, selen

- Signs and symptoms of pancreatic cancer include unintentional weight loss, loss of appetite, abdominal pain, and depression. If you are over 70 and have had such symptoms see your physician. Notwithstanding, the five-year survival rate for pancreatic cancer is a bleak-- 7% and, always with optimism, treated with a multidisciplinary approach.

Breast Cancer—

Men CAN get breast cancer. Men over sixty should react to a painless lump or puckering of the skin around the nipple sometimes accompanied by a bloody discharge and should seek medical attention. Such concern is especially so if the BRCA 1 or 2 gene runs in the family. A history of obesity, prior radiation, abnormal oestrogen levels from liver disease, or alcoholism, are significant risk factors.

It is acceptable to gain 10 to 20 pounds from your nubile high school weight. But remember, that your weight can be deceptive, fat weighs less than muscle. Unsure? calculate your body mass index (BMI), a person's weight in kilograms or pounds divided by the square of their height in meters or feet. Obesity increases all-cause morbidity and incalculable cost to society. A question that haunts me is whether we not be more aggressive treating the obesity epidemic, or continue to pay many millions of dollars for hip, knee, and ankle replacements, the result of weight-related bone and joint destruction.

The Silent Disease

"The silent diseases, osteoporosis, and osteoarthritis, are not just a woman's problem. Over 60, vigorous and consistent weight-bearing exercise by either sex protects or slows bone deterioration. Men have bigger bones and fewer hormonal changes, but have a proportionate decrease in absorption of calcium and bone destruction as women. Steroids, alcohol, and smoking accelerate the loss of bone density.

The "wear and tear" of a lifetime, leading to weight-bearing osteoarthritis injury, affects 27 million Americans. "If I knew I would live this long I would have taken better care of my body," is the frequent lament of someone with destruction of shock absorbing cartilage and bones of the hips, the knees, and spine. Non-weight-bearing ageing joints classically in the tips and middle joints of the fingers, do not escape the deterioration, inflammation, and pain of osteoarthritis. Steroids and hyaluronic acid injections into the knees may provide temporary relief, but many wish they had chosen a surgical alternative years earlier. Stem cell injections are not currently FDA approved.

Liver Disease

When we're talking about the liver, we need to assess our intake of alcohol. Under the Dietary Guidelines for Americans 2020-2025, moderate alcohol consumption for men is defined as two drinks a day or drinks 14 a week for men. A heavy drinker may consume as many as 4 drinks a day and up over 14 a week. There are many options for stopping drinking: Alcoholics Anonymous (AA); different levels of drug or alcohol treatment (in or outpatient);or by incorporating a replacement behaviour like exercise, changing lifestyle, who you associate with, and where you socialize. That is how I gave up smoking 40 years ago and drinking 16 years ago

Screening for substance abuse of any kind should be an integral part of all yearly physicals. The most common screening tool for substance abuse, the CAGE questionnaire, can be helpful: (1) Are you trying to **cutdown** (2) People are **annoying** you by criticising your drinking? (3) Have you felt bad or **guilty** about your drinking? and, (4) Have you ever had a drink first thing in the morning (**Eye Opener**) to steady your nerves or get rid of a hangover?

Excessive alcohol use leads first to a reversible fatty liver or, if chronic, irreversible cirrhosis. Orally developed hepatitis A is usually not lethal; whereas, hepatitis B and C, from contaminated needles or unprotected sex, may lead to dangerous liver damage and failure. Thinking of sex with a new partner? Remember, you are never too old for an STD that are uncomfortable but, ones like HIV or syphilis, can kill you.

Taking Care of Your Teeth

Although I have issues around the availability of dental care for the underserved poor and elderly, I have praise for a dentist's commitment to preventative care, even though their income derives from hygienics, crowns, caps, root canals, repairing, filling, and extracting teeth.

Find a dentist attuned to dental problems for men over 60 such as dealing effectively with ageing cracked teeth and advancing gum recession, your mouth's worst enemy. Sign up for a supplement to Medicare that includes at least minimal dental coverage, especially, if you are living on a modest social security income. Or choose a dentist with an in-house insurance plan you can prepay for discounted benefits for root canals, crowns, fillings, repairs for cracked teeth, and other hazards of ageing.

Flossing is as important for someone over sixty as it is for younger men and women. Regular flossing after meals and before bedtime, carefully manoeuvring between wider spaces between your teeth, can prevent plaque build-up, cavities, or further gum recession. Dentists advocate at least twice-a-year cleaning to effectively remove plaque leading to infected gums and recession.

Men over 60 who have been smokers and drinkers must face demons of the mouth that include damaging periodontal disease or, worse yet, mouth or throat cancer. Smokeless tobacco and pipe smoking combined with alcohol increase vulnerability to oral cancer. Dentists should do a very thorough examination of the mouth at each hygiene appointment. In the event you notice a new tissue change in your mouth, throat, or tongue, that is suspicious, treatment ranges from a short period of observation or, if enlarging, a biopsy.

Oral cancer is divided into two categories. (1) Cancers affecting the lips, teeth, gums, the front two-thirds of the tongue, and the roof of the mouth; and (2) Cancers affecting the oropharynx and the middle part of the throat including the vocal cords. It's time to contact the dentist or personal physician if you notice a persistent white or red patch or sore in your mouth that won't heal, unexplained bleeding, a problem swallowing, a lump in your neck, or persistent hoarseness.

There are 200,000 new cases a year of oral squamous cancer, resulting in 10,300 deaths yearly. With early detection, the five-year survival rate from localized squamous carcinoma of the mouth is %93% but, with lymph node metastasis, the five-year survival rate drops to half Once the cancer has spread to distant organs, the survival rate drops to 33% Surgery varies with the stage of a lesion ranging from a limited excision to wider surgery of lymph nodes, part of the tongue, or even part of the jawbone.

Skin Cancer

Skin cancer is the most common of all cancers but – with one exception, melanoma – usually has a favourable outcome. Skin cancer occurs more frequently if you have been sunburned as a child, are fair-skinned, or spent most of your working and recreational life out-of-doors. Don't overdo the sun and that includes tanning beds. In the sun a lot, apply sunscreen of SPF 30 or more.

Basal cell and squamous cell skin cancers are the most common skin cancers but, fortunately, the least dangerous. Skin Cancer Foundation reports that "At least one in five Americans will develop skin cancer by the age of 70". Squamous and basal cell skin cancers can appear crusty, scaling, itchy, or bleed. Diagnosis depends on the results of a punch, shave, or excisional biopsy. The pathology report determines the next steps.

Squamous, and basal carcinomas rarely spread beyond outer skin layers. Once removed, basal and squamous skin cancers do not usually reoccur in the same location, but are more likely to occur in other sun-exposed places. But they can hide elsewhere.

The great white shark of skin cancers is melanoma. Relatively rare and considered hereditary, melanoma is the most dangerous of the skin cancers, and starts in the pigment-producing melanocytes in the skin. In 2017, there were 87,110 cases with 9,730 deaths. Early diagnosis is vital.

Making a diagnosis of melanoma applies to any suspicious skin change with a lesion larger than a pencil eraser, of mixed colors (red, purple, or black), an asymmetric border, or increasing in size. A physician will determine the next steps if the shave, punch, or excisional biopsy, confirm that your skin change is a melanoma.

Make sure your personal physician or dermatologist looks over all your body at your physical. This is not a time to be modest. The physician must look between your toes and every place the sun never shines. The biopsy must ensure the borders of any specimen are free of melanoma. A melanoma can arise even in those with dark skin. Reggae star, Bob Marley, a dark-skinned Jamaican, died from a melanoma that began between his toes.

Melanoma starts in the top two layers of the skin, the epidermis and dermis, and spreads into the subcutaneous tissue, adjacent lymph glands, and to the liver, lungs, and brain. Treatment runs the gamut from radiation, adjuvant chemotherapy, to immunotherapy.

In summary, many of the physical challenges that men over 60 face can be prevented or changed by adopting and maintaining healthy lifestyles. I recommend less worry or fear, but more proactive and healthy decisions that can ensure achieving a better life after 60. The message I give is to anticipate and accept, inevitable physical and emotional challenges to our bodies. By taking this positive and optimistic approach, I believe we can reduce unnecessary premonitions or fear of death, of immobility, or loss of independence should infirmity threaten the quality of our life over 60. This medical overview provides facts that afford a better understanding of what is avoidable and correctable with a heathier lifestyle; from what is not. Act early and not later. Seek a most qualified and age savvy physician. Expect and demand compassionate health care from those who understand older men but, especially, ensure that the physician you choose honours your strength and potential as a man entering a still vital and exciting time of his life.

Epilogue
Summing Things Up

Be optimistic not fearful about ageing. Fight the challenges of the physical and cognitive transformation of ageing by defying societal stereotypes. Savour aloneness not loneliness. Let spiritualty in. Communication is the secret for loving sex. Prepare for the realities of retirement. Pre-emptively react to correctable health risks as provided. Enhance strength, power, flexibility, and endurance. Joyously exercise and stretch. Make good eating choices. Develop strong support and avoid isolating. Eliminate bad and adore good memories. Catch the sunrise and don't ignore or fear the sunset. Reject uninformed stereotypes. Find support for grief and aloneness. It is what I am now – my gold – not just what I was.

> "There is no way of pretending. Your eyes give you away.
> Something inside you is feeling like we said all there is to say.
> Her imagination ran wild. Could this really be happening to me."
> – Breakdown Tom Petty and the Heart Breakers

An unexpected encounter with an older friend at a favourite local coffee shop brought some final thoughts about the challenges we face as we pass 60. He looked up from where he sat unobtrusively in the back corner of the café. Bob, a retired biologist and college professor who, twenty years prior to retirement, had switched careers to become a medical detective for the state health department.

Bob smiled back at me. It was quite some time since we had shared stories about our lives. I asked how he was doing and told him how delighted I was to see him again.

"Let's catch up," I said. "A year prior when we visited last, I told you I was writing a book to tell how to deal with the challenges we encounter passing sixty. You shared how in the past year you had lost your wife of 50 years. You explained that you didn't want to embarrass your family looking for a new partner. You said that at that time you had some reservations about looking for someone to do things with."

I remembered that, although he was approaching eighty, he seemed younger than his age, was in good physical shape, and had a twinkle in his eye. He became animated and lit up as he shared with me that he had found a new woman friend. When we had first met at the coffee shop, he did not seem emotionally ready to move on. At the time, he seemed at peace despite having lost his wife and dear partner in the past year. He told me now how he had adapted.

"I have my photography club. It keeps me connected and busy. But now I also do things with my new friend, Barbara, several times a week. She's my age, and widowed as well.'

"You have children, don't you, Bob?"

"Yes, I have three daughters, eight grandchildren, and four great grandchildren," he said proudly.

"Wow!" I thought, he really must have started early.

Choosing what I hoped was a more tactful way to ask, "Remind me, Bob, what's your age?" I have learned this is far better way than asking, "How old are you?")

With a wisp of hesitancy, he responded, "I'm 79."

I took his lead and said, "We're right up there, aren't we?"

This was when I thought I saw fear in his eyes.

"Yes, we are," he said.

We then agreed how time at our age seems to pass so fast.

"I figure I have a good 14 years left," he said.

How did he know that? I wondered. *Better to think positively,* I thought.

Men Over 60: Don't Quit Now! is at once a chance to face the realities of ageing and to discover hidden often unexpected surprises as Bob has done. Bob has undergone a metamorphosis from a half century of what he had described as a beautiful marriage with a partner he loved, and with whom he had children, grandchildren, and great grandchildren. His is a not an uncommon shift after the loss of a dear companion, transient aloneness, but unexpectedly, his openness increased the likelihood of a new and wonderful relationship albeit, occurring in his late 70s.

Bob's journey testifies that a man over 60 has resiliency. I encourage optimism as we adapt to life after 60 rather than fear or hesitancy about developing a new relationship. We ought to work from our gut rather than our brain. Bob – by finding another fulfilling relationship-- has been able to make a healthy change in his life. Why not go happily into the twilight of our lives rather than kicking and screaming into darkness?

I have explained how exercise can attenuate cognitive decline. Making the right cognitive decision where to step, run, or jump outweighs the challenges posed by ageing components of our bodies comprising balance and gait. George Sheehan said the body has a set limit of years. Prostate cancer spelled the end for him but well before he prophesized when he would die, or, in his case, when his body would wear out.

Both Bob and another dear friend and colleague winced when I proposed that that many men over 80 become fragile. "I'm 85 and I'm not fragile," Art, a professor emeritus, and sports guru, proudly told me. Unfortunately, macular degeneration ended his ability to drive. Art's devoted Ethiopian driver dried him off in the morning and picked him up from his university office daily. "The new chief of my department has assured me, I can keep my office until someone else needs it." He finally brought home countless memorabilia and passed on quickly.

He was quick to tell me how he maintained his strength and stamina. Despite a quadruple bypass and his retinopathy impacting his vision, Art quipped, "On the days I still come to the university, I walk a mile or two with Nordic poles on the indoor track." He did not allow physical changes of age impact his personal exercise mantra. Alexander Pope quipped in the poem, "An Essay on Man," "Hope springs eternal". Art put up the good fight until, past 90, his strength left him and, elegantly, he passed on surrounded by his family.

My 92-year-old friend, Robert, a retired baker and widower, dutifully goes to physical therapy to exercise daily. He consistently forgoes the bagels and lox we often enjoy after a morning prayer meeting called a minyan. "I can't exercise on a full stomach," he tells me as he moves deliberately for the door in his walker. He and Art have made realistic accommodations so their lives continue to be active and meaningful. Robert, blessed with adequate finances, has a driver as well – more like a personal care attendant disguised as his chauffer. I watch as his driver assists as Bob swings from his walker into the car, yet allows Robert plenty of tether so he can still savour his independence.

When I paid a visit to the third-generation family bakery, there was Robert in a spacious office down the hall from his son, now the CEO. He caught me by surprise as he sat in a white coat and hair net humbly behind a modest desk replete with a monogramed pen set and two or three business periodicals. As we spent an hour chatting and exchanging jokes, I realised that both Art and Robert can maintain freedom that most nursing home residents no longer enjoy.

Another friend, Bill, found maintaining a new relationship unfulfilling. After a year into a new relationship, he perceived his new love interest was not fully engaged in his life due to distractions from her own family. Different yet, similar, his life resembles Robert's, full and content, with different levels of aloneness and personal solutions

Ignore misconceptions society has toward ageing. Society cannot accept that those of us over 60 can still be sexually engaged. Precious little is understood by those around us that retirement can be so painful. I get little slack fearing my own anticipated medical challenges As a retired physician, I know more and fear more. In my medical student and intern days, there were a myriad of "intern's illnesses" I thought I had. We imagined we had all of them. I still have some of that fear in my senior years.

Gaze positively at hidden benefits; albeit, we may run at a slower speed but, on the positive side, we have longer endurance staying power. Despite the incorrect moniker, "There's no fool like an old fool," we have the wisdom of an elder. We have sexual resiliency. Ours can be satisfaction of a life fulfilled and not one of despair that we have not lived a full life or not done enough. This is it, folks. Our lives are not a dress rehearsal. Be advised, my fellow travellers, we HAVE contributed and, as parents, grandparents, friends, and co-workers, we can continue to do so. This is our legacy. We should identify and savour our gold and how we contributed so much to society.

Men Over 60: Don't Quit Now! describes an array of illnesses that may abruptly change the course of our lives. Importantly, they should be faced as if we were duelling as if we were a champion Hungarian fencer. The book explains how early identification of risk factors and red flags may delay or prevent the progression of medical or emotional invaders. Seek the advice of physicians who recognise viability rather than chronological age.

Men Over 60: Don't Quit Now! has laid out realistic possibilities to enhance strength and power, aerobic sustainability, and a wonderful endurance capacity. Continue or begin techniques described in this book to improve your flexibility. Stretching can avoid ripping or aggravating muscle, tendon, or ligament injuries. Making good nutritional choices will nourish efforts to maintain the other ingredients for staying happy and fit over 60.

Dr Marc Agronin, a savvy and erudite Miami geriatric psychiatrist, extols the Harvard seminar he once took with his increasingly age-challenged hero, Erik Erikson. He relates how Erikson's presence was magnificent… he still retained the ability to experience life and interact in meaningful ways with others… although a shadow of his once-renowned acuity. At the limited level he was able to participate, supported by his brilliant wife and collaborator, his presence brought great energy to those fortunate enough to join his coveted seminar. Erikson, in the "Ninth" stage of life – as later defined by his spouse – remained viable albeit no longer capable of remembering but fragments of his lauded accomplishments.

Men Overt 60: Don't Quit Now! offers attainable choices how we, as gray-haired elders, can maintain or even improve our satisfaction and happiness well into "Our Golden Years". Our society has much to gain by recognising how other cultures – unfortunately not always ours-- express appreciation and respect for those of us in retirement. Those who read this book may reassess notions of our value, integrity, and unlimited viability to avoid ill-conceived sadness or despair as we peek surreptitiously around the corner at what comes next.

There is no failure. We did the best we could. We have made a mark on society. Why not explore a renewed or newly discovered spiritualty There is still adequate time to be the best father or grandfather we can. A question an important modality, unfortunately easily overlooked, "Have I had enough fun in my life?" With a bit of reflection, why not recall delightful and comforting memories of crazy antics or embarrassing moment as we hurtled through our earlier lives? Such reflection can make us look at each stage of our lives as if it were a separate book. The time behind us was not a dress rehearsal. It's never too late to STOP counting years, months, weeks, days, hours, minutes, and seconds until retirement. My belief is that it is the human condition to forget the bad memories but relish replace the good ones. "Savour the joy!" Eckhart Tolle advises in the *Power of Now,* the importance of "Living in the present moment and avoiding negative thoughts of the past or fear the future." If you ae undecided how to look back at your life, ditch as many of the bad and painful memories and replace the latter with the wonders of family, friends, and new discoveries.

Reverend Gere in the chapter on *Spirituality Over 60* reflects how we have an awesome presence in the universe and that our children see in us the reflection of the future. It is now for them to take up the torch. Many religions venerate elders. They commemorate the memories of grandparents and parents, understanding that we are part of a flow through generations. Reverend Gere speaks for moving inward with prayer, meditation, and reflection. That is how, he suggests, we may escape the loneliness of ageing. There is inevitable aloneness but there need not be loneliness.

Entering a daily church prayer meeting, a men's group, or a morning minyan as I do – that is a collection of at least ten Jewish men and women, some commemorating a lost father, mother, grandparent, or friend – is a way to openly reconnect with our roots, embedded in spirituality. Gere advises, "Faith communities that live up to the name – churches, synagogues, temples, and mosques – can provide spiritual direction, intellectual stimulation, and moral support while being a touchstone for helping us continually tapping into tradition that touch the core of our being."

As society is ageing, a dwindling work force can offer the opportunity to take unique types of work we never thought we would consider in order stay in touch, challenge the notion of our invisibility; and if physically and mentally capable, work shoulder-to-shoulder with younger workers, and, hopefully, rediscover forgotten invulnerability. Take a chance. Have fun. But also make good cognitive decisions realising the impact visual, proprioceptive, and vestibular decrements to balance and gait have on our day-to-day movements.

It makes more emotional sense to visualise past success rather than to imagine we have failed. In *The Prophet*, Kahlil Gibran explains, "Your children are not your children. They are the sons and daughters of life's longing for itself." Although for me not always easy, it is important to accept the direction my children have taken. Gibran describes how we shoot the arrow into the air but have no control where it may land. Just as we as parents may have limited control of our children's destiny, no one provided a course in parenting. We did the best we could.

We age differently over time. My fiftieth college reunion confirmed that. How we feel about our journey into our late sixties, seventies, and eighties varies. That day in the café, I saw both rekindled spirit but also angst in Bill's eyes. He knows the math defining his longevity. As we pass the 60s mark, we are faced with different joys, successes, failures, and triumphs. I always look to the billowing clouds for sustenance. When I run or ski, I like to feel the mist, the rain, or the snow against my face. Once again, check out the sunrise and don't ignore the sunset. Ride the wave. Savour the tastes, the smells, the closeness, and enjoy every day individually.

Many men and women also define "Who I was" by "What I did day-to-day". Many of us – myself included-- struggle with retirement. Erikson explains that, at 70, he looked back as he did with assistance in that Harvard seminar, but struggled to recall the many books he had written. At our fiftieth college reunion, a survey asked, Had we accomplished everything we had set out to do, and to make our lives count. Many classmates conceded they had accomplished, "Not so much, but I hope I have made an impact on the people I have touched –

my grandchildren, my children, and those others I have known along the way." A questionnaire at the reunion asked. "What would you do differently, if you could do it again?" My answer was a succinct, "I can't." The point is that we cannot do it again, so it is vital to appreciate our vantage point in our lives. Let's call it wisdom.

Men Over 60: Don't Quit Now! has taken us on a journey about the reality of ageing; the misconceptions as well as the vital ingredients that will allow us to view our lives from a perspective of hope. This book has offered strong advice how we can and should refute ageism. Society wants to believe that, just because we are over 60, we should, "Take it easy." "Act your age." My advice is, "DON'T!" Get out there and challenge actuarial statistics. Reject less enlightened stereotypes many attach to ageing. The chronology of our lives has changed. What was once seventy-five can, with the right attitude and activity and lifestyle, be fifty or younger!

As an elder myself, in *Men Over 60: Don't Quit Now!* I have told my readers to savour this part of our lives, and make the most of our unrecognized vitality. This book has emphasised how best to cope with the fear of death, declining physical ability, loss of muscle mass and cardiac capacity, balance and gait changes, cognition, as well as issues of loss and grief.

I hope that *Men Over 60: Don't Quit Now!* enlightens and makes the inevitable less fearful but, both exciting and fulfilling.

Before he removed my cataracts, another long-time friend, an ophthalmologist, reassured me that – despite he is 76 – when most surgeons retire – he saw no reason that his age should or would compromise his ability. He was proud to share that his batting average repairing cataracts was a 100%. Practice more, worry less. Anticipate – or let us call wise choices active cognition. Look before you jump. Make realistic decisions. By tempering enthusiasm with reality, we can prevent falls or other debilitating injuries.

I am heartened. I may take longer, but I'm getting better. There is the bitter and there is the sweet. In almost any sport, by adhering to a regular exercise schedule, we can excel among other competitors our age. That is what age classes in competition are all about, to encourage not to discourage. I am a brown rice and beans guy. With more than 60% of the American population overweight and plenty obese, it is as vital as we pass the 60 mark, to maintain sensible eating habits. Appropriate weight for our age and height helps us get more enjoyment from sport, sex, and retirement.

In retirement, a loss of routine and work friends can affect our sense of purpose. Do not let it. Now is not the time not to be like leaves in the fall; that is, we too dry up and blow away. Leaves at the peak of their color are devastatingly beautiful. Why not take a quiet lull in the backyard hammock between gardening, writing, or exercising? One dear friend anticipates his days caring for his granddaughter. Are these times he missed with his own children? Who cares? Go at it but, perhaps, rejoice that you can do it better this time around.

As men, we easily may define ourselves as, "What I do" or "What I did" to identify "Who I was or am". Unfortunately, this conviction runs deep in our sinews. "I am the person I am." Understanding who we really are takes a little work to find a honest identity? After my father's death and then living in a retirement community, my mother, a retired physician, opined, "No one knows who I am any longer."

She – like so many of us after retirement – may lose what we see as our identity. But, far worse, we can but should not lose the meaning for being. We must honour our self-worth, despite minimising generalisations by society. *Men Over 60:Don't Quit Now!* by exploring unexpected avenues for maintenance and growth, supports healthy self-actualisation combined with a hearty self-esteem.

A hardy sexual and loving relationship can be a thrust for life itself. We still have the juices for love albeit, we are no longer "hound dogs". Emotional struggles are as much a part of our years over 60 as they were in our challenging 40s. My friend and attorney, now over 90, forges ahead. He tells me he reads the Sunday obits as I do looking for friends who have passed. Similar to my café friend, a brief effort to start a new relationship was unsuccessful, and he now relishes his aloneness.

Another dear friend and colleague I spoke about, described how he made several attempts toward another relationship after his beloved wife of 30 years died. He too left the dating arena when he realised "She just didn't listen or seem interested in what I had to say". He enjoys a busy retirement as a mentor to other alternative health professionals. He is healthfully engaged in his adult children's busy lives.

Begin or continue a realistic exercise program. Find a physician who is both in shape and at peace with him or herself, and who says, "You don't look or act 60." After seeking a discriminating physical, just DO IT. This book has explained how to exercise smartly whether you chose to go it alone, in groups of all ages, or in classes at the senior centre. Make exercising joyous not drudgery.

Know your limitations, but do not sell yourself short. Yes, you are slower. But be aware that masters level competition is age specific. Still, as a competitive cross-country ski racer, one of the rewards of passing the 75-year-old mark is being the youngest and strongest in my age group, I am now top dog. Know when it is vitally important to survey the playing field. realistically evaluate if the day is too hot, too dry, too humid, or are you pooped from your long hike or swim the day prior? Listen to your body, but do not overly pamper it because you are over 60 and erroneously listen to those advocating ageist caution.

Men over 60: Don't Quit Now! has explored a multitude of hidden challenges of ageing past 60-- the fears, the joys, and a reawakened spirituality of whatever flavour we cherish. Ageing includes inevitable aches and pains. This may be a time to rediscover sex with a loving mate of over 30 years. It is never too late to learn partner communication skills that can enhance our relationship with a partner of 50 years.

The 60s and beyond can and should be a time for a continued joy of life. Age tempers expectations. Engaging in many of the offerings provided in *Men Over 60: Don't Quit Now!* can make life after 60 fulfilling and revelatory. Stay strong even if society believes you have weakened. Adapt as best you can to losing friends and family by developing new support systems. Maintaining connections with active and like-minded folks of any age can be effective for achieving contentment. Now is the chance to cradle a grandchild in your arms. These are years no longer about empire building. They are about maximising joy healthfully

> "For God's anger lasts a moment;
> Devine life is lifelong.
> Tears may linger for a night;
> Joy comes with the day."
>
> — Psalm 30

Appendix 1
Calculating Life Expectancy

According to the latest figures, average life expectancy in the United States is 77.6 years, compared with 75.4 in 1990, as reported in the July, 2022 issue of the Harvard Health Letter. Furthermore, old age begets older age. Today, a 65-year-old American man can expect to live to 81.6; if he reaches the age of 85, he can expect to live to see 90. Women still outlive men—although the gap is closing—but the same demographic pattern holds. Old age adds to life expectancy.

Harvard Health Letter

How long will I Live?

Here are some sites to explore to learn your life expectancy

"Living to 100" Life Expectancy Calculator by Boston University Professor, Thomas Perls, M.D., MPH

Blue Zones Vitality Compass: How do you compare with those who live to 100?

Blueprint Income Life Expectancy Calculator based on NIH, AARP data. Detailed Statistical Analysis of 400,000 from NIH data by Wharton School Professor Dean Foster: Statistics show that the average American will live until 88. Social Security reports that an average American man will live until 83. Also, the longer we live the longer we will live: a 65 year-old will live to 83; An 85 year-old man will live past 90!

Big Life Expectancy Calculator: Another source for aging data.

How Much Money Will I Need After Retirement?

Consult the **New Retirement Planner** or a reputable wealth management company: there are many options how to plan your retirement security

To own annuities: Yes, or No? Are they Good or Bad?

Annuities that are **sold** by insurance brokers, can provide a reliable income stream in retirement. The downside is that if you die too soon, your family may not get your initial money's investment. Through annuitization, your purchase payments (what you have contributed) are converted into periodic payments to you that can last for life.

According to **MarketWatch**: "Buying annuities is when you have an insurance company invest your money and, in return, you receive an income stream for the rest of your life. Annuities can effectively fit into your retirement planning discussions with your financial professional. If you die before you've received all the money you have invested, make sure that your beneficiaries or favourite charities are named as beneficiaries in your will. Social Security is, in fact, an annuity that increases by eight percent every year just by delaying your start date after full retirement age (FRA) of 70. In the event of your death, your spouse assumes your social security income. So, will your ex-wife! There are pros and cons with annuities. Consult your attorney or financial adviser before investing.

Some quick facts from the Bureau of Data Statistics

An older household spends an average of $45,756 per year. That is $3800 per month after taxes on $57,195 gross income—meaning you need to withdraw this amount from your investments for whatever length after retirement you have calculated you will live.

Here is the bad news: The average 60–69-year-old has only $198,000 in their 401K at retirement. No surprise that many of us over 60 have taken on jobs the shrinking younger generation is unable to fulfil (or don't wish to).

Reverse Mortgages: One hears, "I was broke, but, now, with a reverse mortgage, I can stay in my own house until I die. My house is paid off!

In a word, a reverse mortgage is a loan. A homeowner who is 62 or older and has considerable home equity can borrow against the value of his home and receive funds as a lump sum, fixed monthly payment, or line of credit. But, someone who has chosen to have a reverse mortgage has NO loan payments or real estate taxes. The loan balance to a limit, becomes due and payable when the borrower dies, moves out permanently, or sells the home. Best of all, the money you receive for the reverse mortgage is not taxable because it's a non-taxable loan. The advantage of a reverse mortgage is that it converts home equity into available monies to make later life affordable.

Appendix 2
Calculating Life Stress

Stress, Stress, Stress: include family health, deaths or losses, divorce, moving, financial woes, hassles in the workplace, and legal problems.

<u>Stress List</u>

1. Serious Illness in a family member (excluding death)
2. Serious concern about a family member (excluding illness)
3. Death of a family member
4. Divorce or separation
5. Forced to move to a new house
6. Forced to change jobs
7. Been made redundant or unemployable—welcome to corporate America!
8. Feelings of insecurity at work—see above
9. Serious financial trouble
10. Been legally prosecuted

Appendix 3
Dietary Diversity List

The classic food pyramid has been replaced by MyPlate, information available by the U.S. Government Departments of Agriculture and Health and Human Services (USDA and USDHHS) as Guidelines for Selection of a Nutritionally-Sound Health-Promoting nutritional advice. The plan is divided into 5 sections: vegetables, fruits, grains, protein, and dairy. The diet recommends choosing a diet of two-thirds plant products to include whole grains, fruits, vegetables, and one-third animal protein sources.

MyPlate advises limiting fat intake to 25–35% of your overall diet and avoiding fats that harden at room temperature – especially trans fats. Twenty to 35% of your daily calories should be protein. Go lean and mean. Take a pass on the fatty meat. Instead, eat leaner turkey-based bacon and sausage. Make your tacos with turkey. Twenty-five % of calories should be carbohydrate in the grain family, but make it a dense variety that includes such delectables like eight-grain bread, whole wheat noodles, and brown rice.

Dietary Diversity List

1. Dairy
2. Meat
3. Grain
4. Fruit
5. Vegetable

Appendix 4
Depression Indicators

Depression Indicators

What are the signs and symptoms of depression in men?

Different people have different symptoms. Some symptoms of depression include:

- Feeling sad or empty
- Feeling hopeless, irritable, anxious, or angry
- Loss of interest in work, family, or once-pleasurable activities, including sex
- Fatigue, loss of energy, listless
- Not being able to concentrate or remember details
- Not being able to sleep, especially early awakening, or sleeping too much
- Overeating, or not wanting to eat at all
- Thoughts of suicide or, worse yet, suicide attempts
- Aches or pains, headaches, cramps, or digestive problems
- Inability to meet the responsibilities of work, caring for family, or other important activities.
- Weight loss or gain. Not hungry or too hungry but unrelated to diet
- Feelings of worthlessness
- Diminished ability to think or concentrate, indecisiveness
- Recurrent thoughts of death or ideas about suicide
- Psychomotor agitation – fidgeting, moving, or speaking more rapidly; or psychomotor retardation – moving or speaking more slowly than usual

Appendix 5
Ways to Prevent Neck Pain and Cervical Kyphosis of Ageing

These are great exercise you can do while sitting or standing. The goal is to work on stacking your cervical vertebrae, so they are in as neutral position as possible. This exercise described in the stretching chapter has been a lifesaver for me.

It is not unusual with age that our cervical vertebrae begin leaning forward so that we begin to have rounded shoulders, and we look forward and down. Also, many have degenerative arthritis. When our vertebrae compress, pressure is placed on nerve roots emerging from the disc facets. Shifting a relaxed stack of vertebrae opens up the spaces between the facets and is a welcome alternative to more aggressive and invasive epidurals or painkillers of varied intensity. Sit up straight. Then pull your chin back trying to make a double chin. Concentrate that your head and spine neither flex nor extend. Keep it flat. Now slide your chin forward against a tight fist against the wall taking care not to flex or extend your neck. Put a fist between the back of your head and the wall and feel the bones slide. Repeat this exercise on both sides of your head and you are well on your way to naturally eliminate annoying neck pain.

As we age, we may tilt our heads down and forward while rounding our shoulders. A few simple exercises can prevent this. Are men looking toward the ground to avoid falling? Techniques include Chin Tucks and Juts; stacking cervical vertebrae in a neutral position; Wall Tilts working the lower back, gluts, and core; Wall Arm Circles, like wall tilts, but now your back is flat against the wall, then circling arms against the wall; Scapular Tucks using a resistance band to pull your shoulder blades inward; and the bird dog, a yoga position on your hands and knees strengthening neck and core.

1. **Wall Tilts**:

    Surprise, two for one. This terrific exercise also strengthens your pelvis and gluteal muscles – another technique to relieve nasty low back pain and do some posture work. A roller works well here as well. Stand with your back to the wall. Lay a flat hand behind your lower back and while pulling in your abdominal muscles, tuck in your pelvis. The idea is to flatten your lower back. The tipoff is you will feel pressure against your hand. Careful to keep your shoulders and the back of your head against the wall. Sitting works as well.

2. **Wall Arm Circles**:

If you have mastered the wall tilt, it is time to progress. Start standing again with your back against the wall. This is a combo manoeuvre: walk out six inches or so from the wall. While you feel the wall against your lower back, tuck in your pelvis once again so your lower back lies up against the wall. Get tough; bring your shoulders and head back against the wall. Feeling better? Now for another twist to this exercise. Slowly raise your arms overhead but keeping them consistently against the wall. A challenge? No cheating. After bringing both hands together overhead, bring them back to where you started.

3. **Scapular Retractions**

Here is a chance to throw in a resistance band. No need to get the stiffest. Keep it fun. Loop this instrument of torture around an immovable pipe. A loop in each hand and standing up straight, increase the tension with your arms extended and parallel to the floor. Pull your shoulder blades together. You are getting there: another step for improved posture.

4. **Bird Dogs**

Get down on your hands and knees. What, I did not sign up for a yoga class!

Face down and look at the floor. Keep your head loose, relaxed, and in a neutral position. Suck in your gut to stabilise and straighten out your back.

Now, let the fun begin. Lift and extend one leg so it extends behind you. Lift your opposite arm and likewise extend it in front of you. Straight back now, and do not arch your back. Hold for a few seconds. You can have a friend help you maintain this balancing act. Now lower your leg and arm and go for it again with your opposite arm and leg.

Do not fret. If the combo arm and leg is too difficult, just lift either your arm or leg progressively as you become comfortable with versions adding the opposite leg or arm slowly as you develop balance. This is about progress not perfection.

References

1.A Mark Clearfield, R. Friedman, *JAM Geriatric Society*, 1985 Nov; 33 (11):773–8.

2. Sanjay Sharma, Ahmed Merghani, Luis Mont, *European Heart Journal*, Volume 36, Issue 23, 14 June 2015, Pages 1445–1453.

3. Calculate Life Expectancy with Living to 100, the Blue Zones, Vitality Compass, or The Longevity Tool by Wharton School Professor, Dean Foster,

4. U.S. Department of Agriculture and U.S. Department of Health and Human Services. Dietary Guidelines for Americans, 2020–2025. 9th Edition. December 2020. Available at DietaryGuidelines.gov.

5. Social Security Actuarial Life Table: The current life expectancy for U.S. in 2021 is 78.99 years, a 0.08% increase from 2020. The life expectancy for U.S. in 2020 was 78.93 years, a 0.08% increase from 2019.

6. *The Kominsky Method*, starring Michael Douglas and Alan Arkin, November 16, 2018–May 28, 2021. How I love Alan Arkin now retired from the show.

7. Peter J. Dorsen, M.D., *Dr D's Handbook for Men Over 40: A Guide to Health, Fitness, Living, and Loving in the Prime of Life*, (Wiley & Sons, 2000).

8. Arthur S Leon, M Myers, and J Connett "Leisure-time physical activity and the 16-year risks of mortality from CHD and all causes in the MRFIT," *Intern J. Sports Med.* 18 (Supple 3), Supple 3 1997: 139–254

9. George Sheehan, *Running and Being*: (Rodale Press, 2014).

10. Robert Anderson, *Stretching* (Shelter Publications, Inc. 1975).

Chapter 1 - Fear of Dying

1. *Social Security Actuarial Life Table*: The current life expectancy.

2. "Woody Allen 23 Quotes" (www.GooglescoopWhoopQuotes).

3. Tom Kelly, *Birkie Fever* (Specialty Press Publishers, 1982).

4. Erik Erikson, *Childhood and Society*, (Norton and Company, 1986).

5. Irwin Rosenberg, *The Journal of Nutrition,* V127(5) 1995, May: 9905–9915.

6. P.O Astrand and Irma Rhyming, "A Nomogram for Calculation of Aerobic Capacity (Physical Fitness) from Pulse Rate During Submaximal Work," *Journal of Applied Physiology,* V7(2); 1954: 218–221.

Gianluca, et al. "Acute Subdural Hematoma in the Elderly: Outcome Analysis in a Retrospective Multicentric Series of 21 Patients," *Journal of Neurosurgery,* 49(4); 2020 Oct:

Chapter 2 - Physical Changes of Ageing

1. Deanna L. Huggett, Denise M. Connelly, Tom J. Overend, "Maximal Aerobic Capacity Testing of Older Adults: A Critical Review," *The Journal of Gerontology*: Series A, volume 60(1);January 2005: 57–66.

2. World Health Organization, "Falls," *WHO Global Health Estimates,* 26 April 2021.

3. Peter J. Dorsen, *Dr D's Handbook* for Men Over 40: A Guide to Health, Fitness, Living, and Loving in the Prime of Life, (New York Wylie & Sons 1999): pp 2–7.

4. Aaron L. Baggish, Malissa J. Wood, Athlete's Heart and Cardiovascular Care of the Athlete Scientific and Clinical Update, *Circulation,* V123(23); 14 June 2011: 2723–2735.

5.Barry A Franklin, Paul D. Thompson, "Exercise-related Acute Cardiovascular Events and Potential Deleterious Adaptation Following Long-term Exercise Training: Placing the Risks into Perspective – An Update: A Scientific Statement from the American Heart Association," *Circulation,* Vol 141(13); 2020 Feb: 705–736.

6.James H. O'Keefe, et al, "Potential Adverse Cardiovascular Effects from Excessive Endurance Exercise," *Mayo Clin Proc,* V 87(6); 2012 Jun: 587–595.

7.Benedetta Bartoli, et al, "Age and Disability Affect Dietary Intake," *The Journal of Nutrition,* V 133(9;) 2003 Sep: 2868–2873.

8.William P. Meehan, et. al, "Relationship of Anterior Cruciate Ligament Tears to Potential Chronic Cardiovascular disease," *AmJCard,* V 22(11);2018 Sep 7: 1879–1884 (Also, as the Harvard Medical School Football Players Heath Study at Harvard University).

9.Llus Moat, Roberto Elosua, Josep Brugada, "Long-term Endurance Sport Practice Increasing the Incidence of Lone Atrial Fibrillation in Men: A Follow-up Study," *EP Europace,* V 11(1); 2009 Jan: 648–623.

10.Carl Lavie, et al, "Exercise Training and Cardiac Rehabilitation in Primary and Secondary Prevention of Coronary Heart Disease," *Mayo Clinic Proceedings*, V 84(4); 2009, April: 373–383.

11.Ronald Lee Snarr, et al, "Bodyweight Bosu Ball Exercises," *Strength and Conditioning Journal,* V43(3),;2021 June:117–126.

12.Arthur S Leon, "Reducing Ageing-Associated Risk of Sarcopenia," in *Lifestyle Medicine*, James M Rippe (Boca Raton, CRC Press:2019): 1471pp.

Chapter 3 - Cognition

1.J. Eric Ahlskog, et al, "Physical Exercise as a Preventive or Disease-Modifying Treatment of Dementia and Brain Ageing," *Mayo Clinic Proceedings*, V 86(9); 2011 Sept: 876–884.

2.Gary W Small, Parlow-Solomon "What We Need to Know About Age-Related Memory Loss," BMJ 324(7352); 2002 Jun 22: 1502–1505.

3.National Institute on Ageing (NIA) "Cognitive Health: Memory, Forgetfulness, and Aging: What's Normal and What's Not?" Alzheimer and Related Dementias Education and Referrals (ADEAR): Adear@NIA.NIH.gov. 800–438.

4. Marc Agronin, M.D. *How We Age: A Doctor's Journey into the Heart of Growing Old*, (Boston Da Capo Lifelong Books 2012 Mar 6): 320pp.

5.Kai-Xin, Meng-Shan Tam and Jin-Tai Yu, "Comparison Safety and Effectiveness of Cholinesterase Inhibitors and Memantine for Alzheimer's Disease: A Network Meta-Analysis of 41 Randomized Control Trials," *Alzheimer's Res Ther.* 10(126); 2018:126.

6.Arthur S Leon, "Lifestyle effects on Ageing Cognitive Decline," in *Lifestyle Medicine*, ed. James M. Rippe (Boca Raton CRC Press 2019).

7 Frederick K Goodwin, M.D., and Kay Redfield Jamison, PhD, *Manic-Depressive Illness: Bipolar Disorders and Recurrent Depression*, "Treating the Elderly," (New York, Oxford University Press, 2007): p 814.

8.Gil D Rabinovici, M.D., et al., "Executive Dysfunction", *Behavioural Neurology and Neuropsychiatry* V21(3); 2015, June: 646–659.

9.Zawn Villines, "What to Know About Executive Function Disorder," *Medical News Today*, 2019, June 6.

10.Henry Brodaty and Michael H Connors," Pseudodementia, Pseudo-Pseudo Dementia, and Pseudo depression,", *"Alzheimer's and: Dementia,: Diagnosis, Assessment & Disease Monitoring* (Amst) 12(1) 2020, April: 1–23 e12027.

11. Sharon Shively, M.D., PhD, et al. "Dementia Resulting from Traumatic Brain Injury: What is the Pathology?" *Arch Neural* 69(10); 2012, Oct: 1245–1251.

12.Helios Pareja-Galeano, Noria Garabachea, Alejandro Lucia "Chapter Twenty-one:- "Exercise as a Polypill for Chronic Disease," *Prog in Mol Biol Transl Sci;* V135, 2015: 497–526.

Chapter 4 Balance, Posture, and Locomotion
1.Abraham H. Maslow, "A Theory of Human Motivation," *Psychological Review*, 50(4);1943: 370–396.

2.Dawn Sketon, "Why Does Our Balance Get Older As We Get Older?" *Conversation,* October 8, 2015.

3.Barman A, Chatterjee A, Brhide R "Cognitive Impairment and Rehabilitation Strategies After Traumatic Brain Injury," *Indian J. Psychol Med,* 38(3); 2016: 172–81.

4. 3 "Common Eye Disorders and Disease," *Vision Health Initiative* (CDC), Centres for Disease Control and Prevention.

5.Marlene Franzen, "A Longitudinal Study of Knee Pain in Older Men: Concord Health and Ageing in Men Project," *Age and Aging*, V43(2);2014, March: 206–212.

Chapter 5 Speed and Reaction Time
1.Harley Middlebrook, "Running Doesn't Slow Your Running," *Runner's World, 2020 Sept.*

2.Ray C. Fair, "How Fast do Old Men Slow Down," *The Review of Economics and Statistics*, V76(1);1994, Feb: 103–118.

3.Hong Shao, Li-Quan Chen, Jun Xo, "Treatment of Dyslipidaemia in the Elderly," *J. Geriatric Cardiol*, 8(1); 2011, Mar: 55–64.

4.James F. Sweeny, "Physician Retirement: Why it's Hard for Doctor's to Retire," *Medical Economics*, V 96(4); 2019 Feb 25:12–17.

5. Hospital's Ageing Surgeon Program: LifeBridge Health: The Ageing Surgeon Program, A comprehensive, multidisciplinary, objective, and unbiased evaluation of physical and cognitive function for older surgeons (2401 Belvedere Ave, Baltimore, MD 21215: 410–101–9000).

6. K. Anders Ericsson, "How experts Attain and Maintain Superior Performance: Implications for the Enhancement of Skilled Performance in Older Individuals," *Journal of Aging and Physical Activity, V* 8(4);2000, Jan: 366–372. "The experts can then maintain their attained performance level into old age by regular deliberate practice."

7. Jose Marmekira, Mario Godinko, Peter Vogelare "The Potential Role of Physical Activity on Driving Performance and Safety Among Older Adults." *Eur Rev Aging Phys Act*, 6; 2009: 29–38.

Chapter 6 Retirement
1. Erik Erikson, *Childhood and Society*, New York: Norton, 1950. Erikson made his research well known on the Eight Stages of Psychosocial Development.

2. Chloe Zhao, 2020 *Nomadland*, Searchlite Pictures staring Frances McDormand (also producer), and David Straithairn won Academy awards as Best Picture, Best director and Best Actress. The movie *is* based on the book by Jessica Broder, *Nomadland: Surviving America in the Twenty-First Century,* Norton, 2017

3. Jill S. Guadagno, *Ageing and the Life Course: An Introduction to Social Gerontology,* 1999 Boston: McGraw Hill (College).

4. Ayn Rand, *Atlas Shrugged*. New York: Plume, 1999.

Chapter 7 Spirituality
1. Longmen, Tremper. *The Book of Ecclesiastes,* 1998. Print.

2. Zachary Zimmer, I Carol Jagger, and Yashiko Saito, "Spirituality, Religiosity, Aging, and Health in Global Perspective: A Review," *SSM Popul Health* 2, 2016 Dec: 373–381.

3. Lawrence Lepherd, et al. "Exploring Spirituality with Older People, Rich Experiences," *Journal of Religion, Spirituality & Ageing*, V32(4), 2020: 306–340.

4. **David Kaplan**, PhD, LICSW, and Barabara Berkman, DSW, PhD. "Religion and Spirituality in Older Adults," *Merck Manual Professional Version,* last full review March 2021.

5.Helen Levretsky, "Spirituality and Ageing," *Aging Health* V 6(6); 2010: 749–769.

Chapter 8 Invincibility Versus Invisibility
1.Didieu, Anzieu. (1989) *The Skin Ego (Le-Moi-peau)* (Chris Turner, Trans.). New Haven, Yale University Press.

Chapter 9 Sex is Not a Dirty Word
1.Christopher Evans, MD, MPH; Adam Hoverman; et al. "Preexposure Prophylaxes for the Prevention of HIV Infection Evidence Report and Systematic Review for the US Preventive Services Task Force," *Jama* 321(22); 2019: 2214–2230.

2.Grace L. Reynold, Dennis G. Fisher, Bridget Rogalen, "Anal Intercourse: Results from a Qualitative Study," *Archives of Sexual Behaviour*, 44; 2015: 983–995.

3.Anna Muraco, Karen I Fredricksen-Goldsen, "Turning Point in the Lives of Lesbian and Gay Adults Aged 50 and Over," *Advances in Life Course Research*, V 30; 2016 Dec: 124–132.

4.Robin Bell, "Homosexual Men and Women," *BMJ.* V318(7181); 1999 Feb 13: 452–455.

5.Ryn Pfeuffer, "Absolutely Everything to know About Prostate Massage: Did you Know it Can Help With ED, too?" *Men's Health, 2021 Dec 23.*

6.Roger Peabody, "Increasing Diversity of Sexual Experience – Major UK Study," *HIV & Aids – Sharing Knowledge, Changing Lives*, 2013 Nov 30.

7.Michael H Miner, Janna Dickenson, Eli Coleman, E. (2019). "Effects of Emotions on Sexual Behaviour in Men With and Without Hypersexuality." *Sexual Addiction & Compulsivity*, *26*(1–2): 24–41. (Note Eli Coleman, Ph.D., director since 1991 of Institute for Sexual and Gender Health, University of Minnesota (ISGH) and previously called Sexual Attitude Reassessment (SAR) founded 1970). To contact: 612–625–1500, isgh@umn.edu.

8.Jose A Rodriguez, et.al, "Improved Sexual Function After Total Hip and Knee Arthroplasty for Osteoarthritis," *Orthopaedics*, V44(2);2021 Jan: 111–116).

9.Marmko Mornar Jelavik, "Sexual Activity in Patients with Cardiac Diseases" *Acta Clinical Croatica*, V57(1);2018 Mar: 141–148.

10.George Bataille, (Tr. Dalwood Marx) *Erotism: Death and Sensuality*, Chapter 9, "Sexual Plethora and Death," (San Francisco City Lights Books 1957), 94–109.

11.Halwani, Raja, "Sex and Sexuality," *The Stanford Encyclopaedia of Philosophy*, (Spring 2020 Edition), Edward N. Zalta (ed.)

Chapter 10 Loss and Mood Changes in Men Over 60
1. "Mental Health by Numbers," *National Alliance on Mental Illness (NAMI)* (Arlington, VA, 2022. NAMI Help Line: 800–950–NAMI (6264)).

2.Peter J. Dorsen, Paula Clayton "The Diagnosis and Treatment of Depression in Men," *Clinical Advances in the Treatment of Psychiatric Disorders* V5(1); 1991 January/February.

3. NIH Scientists and other Experts, "Depression and Older Adults," *NIH National Institute on Ageing* (NIA) (NIH Baltimore, MD; 2021, July). National Suicide Prevention Lifeline: 800–273–4727; Substance Abuse and Mental Health Services Administration: 877–726–4727, Samhsain.info@Samsha.hhs.gov.

4.Pim Cuijpers, et al, "Psychological Treatment of Depression in Primary Care: Recent Developments," *Curr Psychiatry Rep*, 21(12); 2019 Nov. 23:129.

5 "Depressive Disorders," *Mayo Clinic*. Current referral literature.

6.Jane Fermestad-Nolp, et al, "Characterological Depression in Patients with Narcissistic Personality Disorder," *Nord J Psychiatry*;73(8); 2019 Nov: 539–545).

7.Sarah Wadd, and Maureen Dutton, "Accessibility and Suitability of Residential Alcohol Treatment for Older Adults: A Mixed Method Study." *Subst Abuse Treat Prev Policy*, 2018; 13(49): 1–9.

8. Shalini Singh, Siddarth Sarkar "Benzodiazepine Abuse Among the Elderly," *J Geriatr Ment Health*, 2016 V3 (2); 2016: 123–130.

Chapter 11 Stretching
1.Daryl J. Cochrane "Alternating Hot and Cold-Water Immersion for Athletic Recovery," *Phys Ther in Sport*, ``V5 (1); 2004 Feb: 26–32.

2. Francoise Bieuzin et al, "Contrast Water Therapy and Exercise Induced Muscle Damage: A Systematic Review and Metanalysis," *PLoS One* 8(4); 2013 April.

Chapter 12 Strength Training

1. I.-Min Lee "No Pain No Gain Thoughts on the Caerphilly Study: Greater Duration and/or Intensity of Activity Can Bring Additional Heath," *Br J Sports Med* 38(1); 2004; Feb: 4–5.

2. Swanson, S, and R. J. Moffatt. 1986. "The Effects of a Strength Conditioning Periodization Program on Muscular Development," National Strength and Conditioning Association, New Orleans, Louisiana.

3. Brent Hamar, DDS, MPH, et al, "Impact of a Senior Fitness Program on Measures of Physical, and Emotional Health, and Function," *Popul Health Manag,* 16(6); 2013 Dec.1; 364–372.

4. Seladi-Schulman, PhD (Rev by Shilpa Amin, MD) "Medicare and Silver Sneakers," *Health Line,* Updated April 15, 2021.

5. Dori E Rosenberg, PhD, MPH, et al, "Barriers to and Facilitators of Physical Activity Program Use Among Older Adults," *Clin Med & Research,* V 12(1–2); 2014 Sept 1: 10–20.

6. Frederick C. Hatfield; March Krotee, *Personalized Weight Training for Fitness and Athletics: From Theory to Practice.* (Kendall Hunt Publishing Company, 1984).

7. Victor L Katch, Frank I Katch, R Moffatt, et al, "Muscular Development and Lean Body Weight in Body Builders and Weightlifters, *Medicine and Science in Exercise,*" V12 (5); 1980 Jan 1: 340–344.

8. Jean Claude Killy with Al Greenberg, *Comeback.* New York: Macmillan/McGraw Hill 1974. Killy won the overall first World Cup in 1968 and the Triple Crown of downhill skiing: downhill, giant slalom, and slalom in the 1968 Winter Olympics in Grenoble, France. His accomplishments range from car racing, movies, ski area building, and running.

9. William J Evans "Resistance, Exercise, Ageing, and Weight Control," 147–165; Lorelee L. Stock, et al. "Resistance Training and Musculoskeletal Injury," 165–181; and Maria Afiatarone-Singh "Elderly Patients and Frailty," 181–215, eds. James E Graves, Ph.D. and Barry Franklin, Ph.D. (Champaign, Ill, Human Kinetics, 2001): 417 pp.

Chapter 13 Aerobic Exercise

1. June Kloubec "Pilates for Improvement of Muscle Endurance, Flexibility, Balance, and Posture." *Journal of Strength Conditioning Research* 2010 March; V24 (3); 2010 March: 661–667.

2.Pete McCall "Hitting the Barre: Understanding the Popular Group Fitness Trend." *ACE Sponsored Research*, 2019 December: 1–3.

3.Joe Miller "ACSM Exercise and Weight Loss Guidelines," *AZ Central*, May 5, 2022.

4.Harsh Patel, et al, "Aerobic Versus Anaerobic Exercise Training Effects on the Cardiovascular System," *World J Cardiol*, V 9(2):;2017 Feb 26:134–138.

5.Mayo Clinic Staff "Exercise Intensity: How to Measure It. Get the Most Out of Your Workouts by Knowing How to Gauge your Exercise Intensity," *Health Lifestyle Fitness*, 2022

6.Lasse Gliemann. "Training for Skeletal Muscle Capillarization: A Janus-faced Role of Exercise," *Eur J Appl Physiol* V 116; 2016: 1443–1444.

7.Robert Bogard. "Athlete's Heart" *Heart* 89(12); 2003 Dec:1455–1461.

8.Yehia Fanous, and Paul Dorian "Wearables for Cardiac Monitoring in Athletes; Precious Metal or Fool's Gold," *European Heart Journal/Digital Health* 2021 Sept; V2(3); 2021 Sept: 358–360.

9.Wendy Bumgardner "Resting Heart and Fitness," *Very Well fit* 2021 October 12.

10. Christine Maslach, Michael Pleita, "Understanding the Burnout Experience: Recent Research and its Implication for Psychiatry," *World Psychiatry, V15(2); 2016 Jun: 103-111.*

11.Nia Mitchell, et al. "Obesity: Overview of an Epidemic," *Psychiatr Clini Nor Am,* V34(4) 2011 Dec;: 717–732.

Chapter 14 An Ounce of Prevention

1.Laura Quaglio. "19 Signs of Overtraining: How to Avoid Excess Fatigue and Overtraining Syndrome (OTS)," NASM.org.

2.Flavio Adssuara Cadegiani, et al. "A Diagnosis of Overtraining Syndrome: Results of the Endocrine and Metabolic Response on Overtraining Syndrome Study: EROS-Diagnosis," *J Sports Med* (Hindawi Publ Corp) 2020 April 22; 39378.

3.Arthur S. Leon "Physiological Interactions Between Diet and Exercise in the Etiology and Prevention of Ischaemic Heart Disease," *Annals of Clinical Research* 20; 1988:114–120.

4. Cameron C. Banks, M.D., John S. Hayward, James A. Wilkerson, Editor, *Hypothermia, Frostbite and Other Cold Injuries*. Seattle, WA The Mountaineers 1986: 105 pp.

5.American College of Sports Medicine, *Guidelines for Exercise Testing, and Prescription 3d ed,* Philadelphia, Lea and Febiger, 1986: 177pp.

6.American Heart Association "American heart Association Recommendations for Physical Activity in Adults." *AHA* 2021.

7.Christopher J. Keating, et al. "Comparison of High-Intensity Interval Training to Moderate-Intensity Continuous Training in Older Adults: A Systematic Review," *Journal of Aging and Physical Activity,* V 28(5); 2020 Apr: 788–807.

Chapter 15 Balancing Aerobics and Strength Training

1.George Sheehan *On Fitness*. New York, N.Y. Touchstone, Sept. 1984: 256 pp.

Chapter 16 Nutrition: You Are What You Eat

1.Henry Blackburn "Invited Commentary: 30-Year Perspective on the Seven Countries Study," *American Journal of Epidemiology,* V185(11); 2017 June: 1143–1147.

2.Arthur S. Leon Part II: Macronutrients; IIB. Micronutrients *Nutrition for Health and Physical Performance*(Course Text), 2015; Kinesiology 5141, University of Minnesota: 1–14

3.Douglas Paddon-Jones, Blake Rasmussen "Dietary Protein Recommendations and the Prevention of Sarcopenia," *Curr Opin Nutr Metab Care* V12(1); 2009 Jan: 86–90.

4. Marcia Hill Gossard, Richard York "Social Structural Influences on Meat Consumption," *Human Ecology Review*, 2003 Summer: V 10(1); 2003 Summer: pp 1–9.

5. Carlo Pinheiro, ed; (Reviewed by Ali Saadoun and Jean-Francis Hocquet), *Front. Sustain, Food Syst*, 2020 October 6.

6. Betty Kovacs Harbolie, M.S, R.D, Author; Melissa Conrad Stoppler, M.D., Medical Editor. "My Plate vs Food Pyramid," *Medicine Net* (medically reviewed 2020 Nov 2).

7. "Dietary Guidelines for Americans," 9th Edition U.S. Department of Agriculture and U.S. Department of Health and Human Services. 2020–2025. Https://www.dietary guideline.gov

8. Louisa Richards (Medically reviewed by Alissa Palladino, MS, RDN, CPT), "Why is Diet So Important for Athletes." *Medical News Today* 2021 April 20.

9. Barbara Strasser, et al. "Nutrition for Older Athletes: Focus on Sex Differences," *Nutrients (Sports Nutrition)* V13(5); 2021:1409.

10. Kirsten Bibbins-Domingo, MD, MAS. "Statin Use for the Prevention of Cardiovascular Disease in Adults US Preventive Services Task Force Recommendations Task Force," *JAMA* V 316(19); 2016: 1997–2007.

11. Ana Diez-Sampedro, et al. "A Gluten-Free Diet, Not an Appropriate Choice Without a Medical Diagnosis," *Nutr Metab*, V 2019; 2019 June: 5 Pages.

Chapter 17 Medical Illnesses Over 60

1. Nicholas H Fiebach, David E Kern, Patricia A Thomas, Roy Ziegelstein, Lee Randol Barker, Philip D Zieve, *Principles of Ambulatory Medicine, Seventh Edition.* Baltimore Wolters Kluwer Health; 2012: 1962 pp.

2. Bruce Leff, Lynda Burton, Scott Mader, John R Burton. "Comparison of Stress Experienced by Family Members Treated in Hospital at Home with that of Those Received Traditional Acute Hospital Care," *Journal of the American Geriatric Society* 56(1); 2008 January: 117–23.

3. John Burton, Samuel Durso, "Dialogue in Geriatrics: How Should We Fix the Problem," *Annals of Internal Medicine* 157(6); 2012 Sept: 455.

4. Arthur S. Leon "Physiological Interactions Between Diet and Exercise in the Etiology and Prevention of Ischaemic Heart Disease," *Annals of Clinical Research*, 20; 1988: 114-120.

5. "Prevalence High Blood Pressure Death from Heart Disease and Stroke Fact Sheet At-a-Glance," *American Heart Association, 2021. www.heart.org/statistics*(Statistics from 2017–2018).

6.Stanley S Franklin "Systolic Blood Pressure: It's Time to Take Control," *American Journal of Hypertension,* V17(53); 2004 Dec: 495–545.

7. "High Blood Pressure Also Known as Hypertension," *National Heart, Lung, and Blood Institute*, Updated May 08, 2020.

8.David Houghton, Thomas W Jones, and Djordje G Jakov "The Effect of Ageing on the Relationship Between Cardiac and Vascular Function," *Mech Ageing Dev.* Jan; V1(53); 2016:1–6.

9.Kathryn K, Garner, MD, William Pomeroy, M.D., James J Arnold, DO, "Exercise Stress Testing: Indications and Common Questions," *Am Fam Physician.* 1:95(5);2017 Sep: 293–299.

10.Jostein Grimsmo "High Prevalence of Atrial Fibrillation in Long-Term Endurance Cross-Country Skiers: Echocardiographic Findings and Possible Predictors-A 28–30 Years Follow-Up Study, "Euro *J Card and Rehab* V17(1); 2919 Feb: 100–105.

11.Eric Bortnick, Conner Brown, et al. "Modern Best Practice in the Management of Benign Prostatic Hyperplasia in the Elderly: *Therapeutic Advances in Urology,"* V12; 2020 May: 1–11.

12.American Counts Staff "2020 Census will Help Policymakers Prepare for the Incoming Wave of Baby Boomers," *2020 Census,* Dec 10, 2019.

13.Juan Rodriguez-Garcia MD, "Radon Gas – The Hidden Killer," *Can Fam Physician* 64(7); 2018 Jul: 496–501.

14.MP Rivera, Richard A Mathay "Passion, Perseverance, and Quantum Leaps: Lung Cancer in the Twenty-First Century," *Clin in Chest Med* V 41(1); 2020 Mar 01: IX–X.

15.Brett C Bade, et al. "Lung Cancer 2020 Epidemiology, Etiology, and Prevention," *Clin in Chest Med* V41(1); 2020 Mar 01:1–24.

16.Justin Sovich, et al. "Colorectal Cancer: Advances in Prevention and Early Detection," *BioMed Research International*, V; 2014.

17.Metn Yelaza, Aydin Inan, Mikdat Bozer, "Male Breast Cancer," *The J Breast Heath,* 12(1); 2016 Jan: 1–8.

18.United Cancer Statistics F(USCS) "Male Breast Cancer Incidence and Mortality US 2013–2017," *US Cancer Stats Data* 2020 Oct.

1.Daniel Morris, Scott Fraser, Christopher Gray "Cataract Surgery and Quality of Life Implications," *Clin Interv Ageing* V2(1); 2007 Mar: 105–108. 1.World Health Organization October 4, 2021.

2.American Heart Association Diet and Lifestyle Recommendations November 1, 2021. "Heart healthy eating patterns."

3.Arthur Leon, co-investigator on many other major NIH funded studies on primary and secondary heart attack prevention, including MRFIT and LRC Coronary Primary Prevention Trial, and the Program on Surgical Control of Hyperlipidaemia (POSCH).

4.Carmen Fiuza-Luces, et al, "Exercise is the Real Polypill," *Physiology* 28 2013: 330–358

5.Physical Guidelines for Americans, 2d edition: U.S. Department of Health and Human Services 2018 Physical Activity Guidelines Advisory Council.

6.Jordon S Querido, A William Sheel, "Regulation of cerebral Blood Flow During Exercise," *Sports Med*, 37(9) 2007;: 765–82

7. Philip N Ainslie, et al, "Exercise improving elasticity of arteries," *J Physio*, 586 Aug. 15: 4005–4010.

8. Jeffrey R Petrella, "Effects of Exercise on cardiovascular risk factors in Type 2 diabetes: a metanalysis" *Diabetes Care*, 34(5) 2011: 1228–1237.

Bibliography

Agronin, Marc E. *How We Age: A Doctor's Journey into The Heart of Growing Old*. Boston: Da Capo Lifelong Books, 2012 320pp.

Anderson, Bob; Anderson, Jean. *Stretching in the 21st Century* (40th Anniversary Edition). Bolinas, CA: Shelter Publication Inc, 2022.

Aronovitch, Jane, Taylor, Mariane, Craig, Colleen. *Get on it! Balance Trainer: Workouts for Core Strength and a Super-Toned Body*. Berkeley: Ulysses Press, 2008.

American College of Sports Medicine. *Guidelines for Exercise Testing and Prescriptions*. Third Edition. Philadelphia: Lea & Febiger, 1986.

Anzieu, Didier. *The Skin Ego.* New translation by Naomi Segal of the History of Psychoanalysis Series, Formerly *Le Moi-Peau*. New York: Routledge Taylor & Frances Group, 1995.

Barker, L. Randol, Fiebach, M. *Principles of Internal Medicine, Seventh Edition.*

Philadelphia: Lippincott Williams& Wilkins, 2007.

Bell, Allan P, Weinberg, Martin S, Hammersmith, Sue Kiefer. *Sexual Preference Its Development in Men and Women*. Bloomington, IN: Indiana University Press, 1981.

Bell, Robin. "Sexual Health of Homosexual Men and Women." *British Medical Journal* V318(7181);1999 Feb 13.

Bennedict, Ruth. *Patterns of Culture*. (New York: Houghton Mifflin Harcourt Publishing Company), 1989 (First edition:1934).

Bly, Robert. *Iron John: A Book About Men*. (New York Knopf Doubleday, 1970).

Boston Women's Health Book Collective. *Our Bodies, Ourselves A Book By and For Women*. New York: Atria Books, 2011).

Bryson, Bill. *A Walk in the Woods*. New York: Doubleday, 1997.

Chopra, Deepak. *Quantum Healing Exploring the Frontiers of Mind/Body Medicine*. New York: Bantam Books, 1989.

Cohen, Leonard. *Book of Longing*. New York: HarperCollins, 2006.

Cooper, Kenneth, H. *Aerobics*. New York: Bantam, 1968.

DeVito, Fred, Halfpipe, Elizabeth. *Barre Exercise You Can Do Anywhere for Flexibility, Core Strength, and a Lean Body*. (Beverly, MA: Fair Winds Press, 2016.

Dodson, Betty. *Sex for One- The Joy of Self-Loving*. New York: Three Rivers Press, 1996)

Dorsen, Peter J. *Dr. D's Handbook for Men Over 40: A Guide to Health, Fitness, Living in the Prime of Life*. (New York: Wylie & Sons, 1999).

Dorsen, Peter J. *Crazy Doctor: Mixing Drugs and Mental Illness*. (Minneapolis, Triple A Press), 2012.

Dorsen, Peter J. *Up From the Ashes: One Doc's Struggle with Drugs and Mental Illness*. (Lavergne, Tenn: Ingram Spark), 2018.

Erikson, Erik H. *Identity, and the Life Cycle*. New York: Norton & Company, 1959.

Erikson, Eric H, Erikson, Kivnick, Q, and Erikson, Joan M. *Vital Involvement in Old Age*. New York: WW Norton, 1986.

Evans, Eric, Loehr, James, Series Editor. *Mental Toughness Training for Cross Country Skiing: Achieve Your Ideal Performance State for Developing Mental Toughness Skills*. New York: The Stephen Greene Press/Pelham Books, 1990.

Fixx, Jim. *The Complete Book of Running* (Second Edition). New York: Random House, 1977.

Franklin, Barry A, Oldridge, Neil B, et al. *Sports Ball Exercise Handbook*.(Originally, *On the Ball*) Second Edition. Monterey: Exercise Science Publishers, 2001.

Frieden, Betty. *The Feminine Mystique*. New York: Random House Publishing House, 1984

Freud, Sigmund. *A General Introduction to Psychoanalysis* (New Translation by Naomi Segal). New York: G. Stanley Hall, (Originally published 1990).

Ibid. *Interpretation of Dreams* (Tr. A.A. Brill). New York: Macmillan, 1913.

Gaby, Alan R. Nutritional Medicine (Second Edition) Concord, NH: Fritz Perlberg, Publishing, 2017.

Goodwin, Frederick K, Jamison, Kay Redfield. Manic Depressive Illness and Recurrent Depression Second Edition. New York: Oxford University Press, 2007.

Gray, John. Me are from Mars Women Are from Venus. New York: Harper Collins Publishers, 1994.

Haas, Robert. Eat to win: The Sports Nutrition Bible. New York: Three Rivers Press, 2000.

Hart, Micky with Jay Stevens. *Drumming at the Edge of Magic a Journey into the Spirit of Percussion*. San Francisco: Harper San Francisco, 1990.

Hatfield, Frederick C. Krotee, March, *Personalized Weight Training for Fitness and Athletics: From Theory to Practice*. Dubuque: Kendall Hunt Publishing Company,1984).

Hicks, Robert. Colorado Springs: NavPress Publishing Group, 1993.

Jameson, J. Larry, Fauci, Anthony, et al. Harrison's Principles of Internal Medicine.(Vol.1 & Vol.2) New York: McGraw Hill, 2018.

Kauth, Bill. *A Circle of Men The original Manual for Men's Support Groups*. New York. Martin's Press, 1992.

Leff, Alan R. ed. *Cardiopulmonary Exercise Testing*. Orlando, Fla: Grune & Stratton, Inc, 1986.

Leon, Arthur S (Ed). *Physical Activity and Cardiovascular Health*. Champagne, Ill: Human Kinetics, 1997.

Levinson, Daniel K. *Seasons of a Man's Life*. New York: Random House, 1978.

Levinson, Daniel K, Levinson, Judy D. *Seasons of a Woman's Life*. New York: Alfred A. Knopf, 1996.

Longmen III, Tremper. *The Book of Ecclesiastes (The New International Commentary on the Old Testament*. Grand Rapids, MI: Eerdmans, 1997.

Maslow, Abraham. *A Theory of Human Motivation*. Psychological Review 1943: V50#4, Pages 370-396.

Ibid. *The Psychology of Science: A Reconnaissance*. New York: Harper & Row, 1966.

McDougall, Christopher. *Born to Run: A Hidden Tribe*. New York: Knopf Doubleday Publishing Group 2011.

Mead, Margaret. *Male and Female: A Classic Study of the Sexes in a Changing World*. New York: Quill (HarperCollins), 1998 edition.

Michaels, Jillian(With Myatt Murphy). *The 6 Keys: Unlock Your Genetic Potential for Ageless Strength, Health, and Beauty*. New York: Little Brown, 2018.

Mothering Magazine (Edited by Anne Pedersen and Peggy O'Mara). *Being a Father, Family, Work, Self*. Santa Fe, Third Printing, 1993. Santa Fe.

Orban, Bill, Nichols, William J, ed. *Royal Canadian Exercise Plans for Physical Fitness*. New York: This Week Magazine, (originally 1961).

Osler, Sir William, Hisae, Niki. *Osler's Way of Life and Other Addresses*. Durham, NC: Duke University Press Books, 2001.

Partin, Allan; Kavousi, Louis R, et al. *Campbell-Walsh-Wein Handbook of Urology*. Cambridge, MA: Elsevier, 2021.

Perelman, Sidney J. *The Road to Miltown or Under the Spreading Atrophy*. New York: Simon & Shuster, 1957.

Price, Joan. *Naked at Our Age Talking Out Loud About Senior Sex*. Berkeley, Ca: Seal Press, 2015.

Ibid. *The Ultimate Guide to Sex After 50 How to Maintain-or Regain-a Spicy, Satisfying, Sex Life*. Jersey City, NJ: Cleis Press, 2015.

Quadagno, Jill. *Aging and the Life Course*. New York: McGraw-Hill, 1999.

Radcliffe, James C; Farentinos, Robert C. *High-Powered Plyometrics*. Champaign. IL, 1999.

Rakel, David P. *Integrative Medicine*, 4th Edition. Cambridge, MA: 2018.

Rand, Ayn. *The Fountainhead*. Indianapolis: Bobbs-Merrill, 1943.

Shahn, Ben. *Ecclesiastes or, The Preacher*. New York: Grossman Publishers and Trianon Press, 1971.

Sheehan, George. *Running and Being. The Total Experience*. Emmaus: Rodale,2013.

Spirduso, Waneen W. Francis, Karen L. Macrae, Priscilla G. *Physical Dimensions of Aging*, Second Edition. Champaign, Ill: Human Kinetics, 2005.

Steinem, Gloria. *Outrageous Acts and Everyday Rebellions*. New York: Holt & Company, 1995.

Strayed, Cheryl. *From Lost to Found on the Pacific Crest Trail*. New York: Knopf Doubleday Publishing group, 2012.

Sweet, Lisa. *365 Sex Positions A New Way Every Day for a Steamy, Erotic Year!* Berkeley: Amorata Press, 2020.

The American Psychiatric Association. Diagnostic and Statistical Manual of Mental Disorders(DSM-5). Washington: American Psychiatric Publishing, 2020.

Tolle, Eckhart. *The Power of Now*. Novato, CA: Namaste Publishing Inc, 2004.

Vanderburg, Helen. *Fusion Workouts, fitness, Yoga, Pilates, and Barre. Champaign. IL:* Human Kinetics, 2017.

Westheimer, Ruth K. *Sex After 50: Revving up the Romance, Passion & Excitement! (The Best Half of Life)*. Fresno, CA: Quill Driver Books, 2005.

Winokur, George; Clayton, Paula J. Limberg; Reich, Theodore. Manic *Depressive Illness*. St Louis: Mosby, 1969.

Lehu, Pierre A.(with). *Sex for Dummies*. Hoboken, N.J: Wiley, 2016.

Westerheimer, Ruth K. *Dr. Ruth's Encyclopaedia of Sex*. Bloomsbury, NJ: Bloomsbury Publishing Plc, 1994.

Wilkerson, James A, Bangs, Cameron C, Hayward, John S. Prevention, *Recognition, and Prehospital Treatment Hypothermia, Frostbite, and Other Cold Injuries*. Seattle: The Mountaineers, 1986. Winston, Sheri. Women's *Anatomy of Arousal Secret Maps to Buried Pleasure*. Kingston NY: Mango Garden Press, 2010.

Glossary

Achilles Tendonitis: The tough fibrous band connecting the strong calf muscles to the heel bone (calcaneus).

Acid Reflux: When stomach acid pushes backward into the lower oesophagus causing nausea or pain. Acid reflux and heartburn more than twice a week may indicate gastro oesophageal reflux disorder (GERD). Symptoms include burning pain in the chest that usually occurs after eating and worsens lying down. Relief possible with lifestyle changes (lose weight, stop smoking, and curtail alcohol and fatty meals), and elevating the head when recumbent. Use over-the-counter medications such as antacids. Histamine 2 inhibitors work in 50%. H2 Proton pump inhibitors decrease acid production more effectively.

Acromial-clavicular (AC) Separation: Varying tears of the ligament connecting the collar bone (clavicle) to the scapular acromial process with or without injury to the coracoclavicular ligament. Some call it a "Piano Key" shoulder injury that can produce pain, instability of the shoulder, and arthritis.

ACSM: The American College of Sports Medicine.

Actinic Keratosis: A precancerous skin lesion usually smaller than a quarter inch, rough, and scaly, varying in color: pink, red, or flesh-colored especially on skin exposed to the sun—the face, ears, back of hands, collar, or nose.

Adult (maturity) Onset Diabetes: Type 2 diabetes, genetic and characterized by high blood sugar, insulin resistance, that is amenable to diet, and exercise-related weight loss that also responds to oral hypoglycemics. Type 2 Diabetes is characterized by massive sugar elevation and associated with hyperosmolar imbalance rather than ketoacidosis as in Type 1 diabetes.

Aerobic Exercise: Exercising efficiently supplying muscles with oxygen

Aerobic Capacity: Maximum aerobic capacity increases with aerobic training. The resting VO_2 is stable, as is the VO_2 at a given workload. The changes are specific to the trained muscles.

All-Cause Dementia: Cognitive deterioration relating to risk factors of age, genetics, head injury, heart disease, stroke, hypertension, or high cholesterol.

Alpha Blocker: A blood pressure medication, an α-adrenoreceptor antagonist, lowers blood pressure by keeping the hormone norepinephrine from tightening the muscles in the walls of smaller arteries that cause high blood pressure.

Alpha-2 receptor Blocker: Alpha-2 blockers or α_2 blockers, are a subset of the alpha blocker class of drugs and are antagonists to the α_2 adrenergic receptor.

Alprostadil: a medication that vasodilates and relaxes muscles and blood vessels that keep blood in the penis that produce an erection. Trade name is Caver jet or Muse either injectable into the penis or by inserting a piece the size of a piece of rice into the urethra.

Alzheimer's (AD): Alzheimer's is a progressive disease. Dementia symptoms gradually worsen over several years. In its early stages, memory loss is mild, but with late-stage Alzheimer's, individuals lose the ability to carry on a conversation or respond to their environment. Alzheimer's is a progressive brain disease that leads to broken connections between nerve cells and tissue shrinkage in parts of the brain essential for memory functions.

Altitude Sickness: Mild to life-threatening physical distress adjusting to lower oxygen pressure at high altitude usually developing between 6 and 24 hours after reaching altitudes more than 2,500 meters above sea level. It presents as headache, nausea, shortness of breath, and loss of exercise strength.

Anaemia: A drop in hemoglobin, hematocrit, red cell indices in a man over 60, unless proven otherwise, may be due to iron loss from polyps a cancer, or a GI bleed anywhere in the bowel. Other causes include inadequate B12, folate, or due to chronic disease.

Anaerobic Threshold: break point when metabolism becomes less efficient, and muscles begins utilizing fats and proteins producing lactate.

Angina: Pain running down the left arm, the cheek, or over the chest from narrowing coronary arteries that increases or decreases, differentiating it from the constant discomfort of a myocardial infarction. Depending on severity, it can be treated by lifestyle changes, medication, angioplasty, or surgery.

Antihistamine: An anticholinergic that includes chlorphenamine and promethazine, commonly used to control allergies and is associated with dry mouth and sedation.

Antioxidants: Attack cancer-causing free radicals by donating an electron to a free radical making it less reactive and harmful.

Antipsychotics: Are neuroleptics that treat a wide range of psychiatric illnesses.

Aphrodisiac: Any substance, behaviour, or substance, such as plants, spices, foods, drink---even money---that may attract or arouse another person.

Apoptosis: Programmed cell death. Unfortunately, occurs all too unavoidably in men over 60.

Arrhythmias: Irregular heartbeats including atrial fibrillation, heart block, and life-threatening ventricular fibrillation or tachycardia.

Asthma: Mild to life-threatening spasm of the muscular pulmonary airways from allergy, infection, pollutants, emotional stress, or cold air producing shortness of breath accompanied by wheezing.

Atherosclerosis: Calcium and plaque build-up in arteries.

Atkins Diet: is a low-carbohydrate fad diet devised by Robert Atkins in the 1970s primarily of fats and proteins that puts people at risk to develop ketoacidosis.

Athletic Heart Syndrome (AHS): Enlarged heart from long-term endurance sports accompanied by bradycardia (a pulse less than 60), that increases blood supply and oxygen to exercising muscles by increasing stroke volume (the amount of blood ejected per beat) with increased chamber size and compliance.

Atrial Fibrillation: the rhythm disturbance described as irregularly irregular rhythm that can compromise exercise level, and may be corrected with medications or ablation of irregular atrial conduction circuits.

Atypical Antipsychotics: The second-generation antipsychotics are serotonin and dopamine antagonists, without the side-effects of the major tranquilizers such as Thorazine (chlorpromazine) or Mellaril (thioridazine) that can over sedate or produce pseudo-Parkinson's called tardive dyskinesia(TD). They are effective for schizophrenia, bipolar disorders, autism, and as an adjuvant in major depressive disorders (MDD). They may have serious anticholinergic side effects like sedation or urinary retention.

Barre: A fun exercise technique derived from classical dance and yoga maintaining joint flexibility, lengthening muscles, improving posture, and overall well-being.

Basal Cell Carcinoma: As with Squamous carcinoma is the most frequently diagnosed cancer and responds to well to varied excisional techniques including MOH's dissection.

Benign Positional Vertigo: Is the sensation of dizziness (vertigo), light-headedness, unsteadiness, loss of balance, sometimes accompanied by nausea when shifting from lying to standing. Correctible by retraining little bones in the semi-circular canals (ossicles) with the Epley manoeuvre.

Benzodiazepine: "Benzos" as they are called, calm and sedate by raising levels of the inhibitory transmitter, GABA, in the brain. They include such overprescribed drugs as Valium (diazepam), Xanax (alprazolam), and Klonopin (clonazepam).

Beta Blocker: A blood pressure pill like Propranolol (inderal) or Tenormin (atenolol) that lowers heart rate and effectively treats chronic congestive heart failure.

Biceps Femoris: One of three muscles responsible for flexion of the knee in concert with the semitendinosus and the semimembranosus. This important and powerful set of muscles called our hamstrings oppose the mighty quadriceps femoris.

Bipolar Disorder: A set of inherited or situational behavioural changes ranging from bipolar 1, associated with mania and depression to bipolar 2, associated with less severe hypomania and similar depression. Medications: Antiseizure medication such as Depakote (valproic acid), Neurontin (gabapentin), Tegretol (carbamazepine), Trileptal (oxcarbazepine), and Lamictal (Lamotrigine), are proven effective.

Black Ice: A dark old sheet of ice sometimes lying under fresh snow that is a fall waiting to happen.

Blood Thinner: Anticoagulant range from a children's 80mg aspirin that decreases platelet adhesivity to heparin, either parenterally; or coumadin (warfarin) orally, to prevent blood clots as in someone with chronic atrial fibrillation or thrombophlebitis. If untreated someone with atrial fibrillation or thrombophlebitis may have an ischemic stroke.

Bone Marrow Transplant: The process of introducing normal stem cells to a suppressed bone marrow that such cells will repopulate and produce normal cells for red and white cell production.

Bosu Ball: A two-sided fitness tool: one side a soft rubber half ball, the other a platform that can challenge and improve balance and improve core strength.

BPH: Benign prostatic hypertrophy that is not cancer but in men over 60 can lead to frequency and obstruction.

Breast Cancer in Men: It occurs! Any physical changes to the nipple or surrounding areola such as puckering, bleeding, and of higher risk in men with obesity or alcoholism.

Buprenorphine: Given IM or sublingual, is a partial agonist-antagonist that prevents withdrawal symptoms either alone or with naloxone, an opioid antagonist.

Buff: Looking hot. Also, a one-piece neck scarf that can cover the whole face.

Burn Out: The result of overtraining and feeling stale, low energy, often with a rapid pulse on awakening.

Burr Holes: Known historically as trephining: holes drilled into and through the cranium onto the brain surface to relieve pressure from a brain bleed, subdural, or epidural hematoma that is either acute or chronic, especially with a palpable fracture and a fixed pupil. Burr holes prevent a great risk of the brain herniating into the base of the brain and spinal cord.

CAGE: A fast assessment to determine alcoholism: Cutdown? Annoyed? Guilty? Eye opener?

Calcaneus: The heel bone to which the Achilles tendon attaches.

Calcium Channel Blockers: Medications like Procardia(nifedipine) and Norvasc (amlodipine) lower blood pressure by blocking calcium, allowing blood vessels to relax to dilate peripheral circulation.

Canadian Airforce Exercises: Five basic exercises (5BX), by Bill Orban in the late 50s to improve the fitness of isolated and deconditioned Canadian pilots in 11 minutes a day.

Cardiac catheterization: Is the gold standard in which a physician runs a special catheter from the wrist or femoral(groin) artery to the heart to evaluate heart wall motion, coronary blood flow, cardiac output, and valve function.

Cardiac Output (CO): The amount of blood the heart pumps per minute.

Cardiac Rehabilitation: Monitored exercise program after cardiac bypass, ablation procedures, or pulmonary problems like COPD.

Cardiolite (Thallium): A cardiac stress test (GXT) with a nuclear tracer demonstrating blood perfusion of cardiac muscle.

CAT Scan: Computerized tomography, a series of x rays of bone, blood vessel, and soft tissue injury.

Cataracts: Age, trauma, genetic predisposition to a chemical change producing clouding of the lens. Effectively treated when an ophthalmologist replaces the lens with a plastic equivalent.

Chlamydia: A bacterial STD detected more in women as a discharge or as dysuria in men.

Calcium Channel Blocker: A blood pressure medication that controls the movement of calcium in and out of cells.

CBT: Cognitive behavioural therapy employs verbal and behavioural techniques helping patients recognize that negative perceptions of themselves are inaccurate.

Cholesterol: The major body fat comprised of high-density lipid (the "good fat") and low-density lipid (the "bad fat).

Clitoris: The small sensitive erectile tissue at the anterior end of the woman's vulva.

Cock Ring: worn around the base of the penis and/or the scrotum to maintain an erection, or recreationally to enhance sexual pleasure.

Core: The strength zone of strong abdominal and back muscles

Cognition: The ability to process and acquire knowledge and understand the process thought, experiences, and the senses.

Cologuard (FIT): Non-invasive immunochemical test of stool for blood. More false positives.

Colorectal cancer: Second largest killer of men over 60.

Colonoscopy: The painless threading of a fibreoptic colonoscope through the large bowel to find polyps or cancer. starting at 45 and then every 10 years unless at high risk and then more frequently.

Colostomy: Surgically diverting the colon to an abdominal opening and a bag.

Complementary amino acids: different proteins in foods like beans and rice complement each other's amino acid pattern to produce complete proteins.

Complex Carbohydrates drinks: Easily absorbed sports drink that is a combination of sucrose, glucose, and dextrose.

Concussion: Mile traumatic brain injury (TBI) with headaches, poor concentration, memory loss, loss of balance, and coordination.

Connective Tissue: Is body tissue that connects, supports, or separates other tissues or organs. Inelastic and after cardiac injury a less effective contribution to heart muscle.

COPD: Chronic obstructive lung disease including chronic bronchitis, emphysema, and asthma.

Corpus Cavernosis: Three blood-vessel rich cylinders in the penis that with arousal fill with blood making an erection.

Corpus Callosum: White matter crossing the midline of the brain and connecting the right and left hemispheres.

Cortisol: The hormone produced by the adrenal gland controlling carbohydrate and other metabolic and hormonal body requirements.

Cowper's Glands: Located just below the prostate producing thick clear mucus prior to ejaculation.

CPC: Clinical pathological conference or when men over 60 take a walk together and talk about their latest medical challenge.

Crunches: Static partial flat or incline sit-ups especially strengthening the upper abdominal muscles.

CT Angiogram: a non-invasive coronary blood vessel calcium scan.

Curls: Strengthening techniques for both upper body biceps and lower hamstring muscles.

DASH Diet: Dietary Approaches to Stop Hypertension emphasizing fruits, vegetables, and low-fat dairy.

Dementia: Impaired memory, judgment with forgetfulness, declining social skills, thinking, and ultimately compromised activities of daily living(ADLs).

Diarthrodial Joint: A joint that only flexes and extends like the knee and elbow.

DNA: Deoxyribonucleic acid is a molecule composed of two polynucleotide chains that coil around each other to form a double helix carrying genetic instructions for the development, functioning, growth, and reproduction of all species. In conjunction with RNA DNA affects gene expression.

ED: Erectile dysfunction.

Ejection Fraction: The ejection fraction is the percentage of blood ejected from a heart with each contraction.

EKG: An electrocardiogram measuring electrical conduction of the heart.

EMR: Patients' electronic medical record.

Endocrine System: Produce hormones beginning with direction from the hypothalamus to target organs like the thyroid and adrenal glands regulating metabolism.

Endothelium: The smooth muscle lining arteries and arterioles.

Epididymis: Transports sperm from the testes to the vas deferens.

Ejaculatory Duct: Delivers sperm into the urethra

Epley Manoeuvre: Techniques to overcome benign positional vertigo.

Essential amino acids: Histidine, isoleucine, leucine, lysine, methionine, phenylalanine, threonine, tryptophan, and valine from food and combining with nonessential amino acids to produce protein.

Executive Function: Thinking processes controlling behaviour and judgment.

Exercise Intensity: The amount of exercise to accomplish a particular activity level.

Exercise Zones: Five levels of activity ranging from under aerobic to and above the anaerobic threshold.

Fast Twitch Muscle: Responsible for speed predominating in younger men.

Ferritin: Iron carrying protein that is reduced in anaemia.

Flomax: Tamsulosin, an alpha blocker, relaxes smooth muscle of the prostate and bladder improving urinary flow for men over 60, especially with an enlarged prostate.

Foreskin: Sheath of skin over the head of the penis.

Free Radicals: Harmful highly charged ions attacked by antioxidants.

Frostbite: Crystallization and blood clots in peripheral vessels.

Frostnip: Ice crystals in the subcutaneous fat. May lead to frostbite.

Gastritis: Increased acid production in the stomach with heartburn.

Glans Penis: The sensitive end of the penis containing the end of the urethra for urine and ejaculate.

Gluteal Muscles: Includes the gluteus maximus, medius, and minimis, "The Butt."

Gluten Intolerance: An immune reaction to eating gluten, a protein found in wheat, barley, and rye affecting the smooth muscles of the small intestine and producing diarrhoea and bloating.

Glycogen: Multibranched polysaccharides that store glucose in the liver and muscles.

GXT: A graduated stress test.

Gynecomastia: Swelling and tenderness of male breast tissue related to puberty, aging, medications, or health conditions that affect testosterone and estrogen.

HACE: High altitude cerebral edema, occurring from 5,000 to 10,000 feet elevation.

HAPE: High altitude pulmonary edema.

Heart Monitor: Chest or wrist detection of pulse and a review of statistics from your workout: elevations, duration, intensity, even location.

Heat Cramps: Dehydration and overall discomfort.

Heat Exhaustion: Worsening response to excessive heat with dehydration and temperature to 103 degrees F with dilated pupils.

Heat Stroke: Life threatening response to excessive and prolonged heat and dehydration with body temperatures exceeding 106 degrees Fahrenheit.

Hemorrhagic Stroke: The result of an exploding arterial blood vessel into the brain.

Hemorrhoids: Congested anal veins: itchy, bleeding, and painful.

Hepatitis: Type A: food born; Type B: Body fluids; Type C: Contaminated needles/sex.

Hierarchy of Needs: Maslow's theory of motivation according to five categories of human needs: (1)Safety/security, Belonging/love, (3) esteem/prestige, and (4)self-actualization/Achievement.

High density lipoprotein: The "Good" cholesterol. Enhanced by exercise.

High Intensity Workouts: Stages 4 and 5 exercise levels.

Hyperparathyroidism: Three-part presentation: "Bones": calcium metabolism and osteoporosis; "Moans": kidney stones; "Groans": emotional problems.

Hypertension: Multiple readings over 120 systolic and/or over 90 diastolic. Related to increased morbidity and mortality from stroke, myocardial infarction, or chronic renal failure.

Hypertrophic Obstructive Cardiomyopathy: Thickening of the heart muscle causing heart failure with shortness of breath, and rhythm disturbances.

Hypoglycemia: Low blood sugar

Hypomania: Less severe than mania and associated with bipolar 2 disorder.

Hypothermia: The result of prolonged exposure resulting in extremely low and potentially lethal core body temperatures.

HIIT: Safe high intensity interval training. Interspersing short bursts of anaerobic with less intense active recovery exercise.

Immunotherapy: Cancer therapy activating or suppressing the immune system.

Isokinetic Exercise: An isokinetic contraction is a dynamic contraction, but the speed of the entire movement is controlled by the exercise machine.

Isometric Exercise: A form of exercise involving the static contraction of a muscle without any visible movement in the angle of the joint such as The Plank.

Isotonic Exercise: Isotonic exercise: Exercise when a contracting muscle shortens against a constant load, as when lifting a weight.

Jogging: A form of running like trotting at a slow and steady pace introduced by Arthur Lydiard from New Zealand in the 1960s and 70s.

Kinesiology: The discipline that studies the mechanics of body movements.

Kyphosis: Excessive forward curvature of the spine: "hunchback" posture.

LADC: Licensed alcohol and drug counsellor.

LDL: The "bad" cholesterol.

Ligament: Short, tough but flexible bands of connective tissue connecting two bones, a cartilage, or binding a joint.

Lipids: Total cholesterol, LDL, HDL), and triglycerides.

LSD: Hallucinogenic lysergic acid diethylamide, "Acid" but also long slow distance training that builds capillarization and oxygenation of lower extremities increasing endurance capacity.

Lubricants: Products that are silicone-based, oil-based, polyunsaturated, and petroleum based to safely lubricate sexual activity.

LVH: Left ventricular hypertrophy also called the "athletic heart" from long term endurance training.

Labia Majora and Minima are sensitive tissue around the vaginal opening. The inner or minima covers the prepuce (hood) of the clitoris and the urethra.

Macular Degeneration: Age-related either wet or dry degenerative tissue in the choroid layer behind the retina at the back of the eye. Leaky fluids of the wet variant with neovascularization build scar tissue around the macula, and if untreated, may lead to blindness. Eye vitamins high in lutein are preventative.

Magnetic Resonance Coronary Angiography: Non-invasive but less sensitive than the "Gold Standard" angiogram.

Mediterranean Diet: A predominantly plant-based diet of vegetables, fruits, herbs, nuts, beans, and whole grains with moderate amounts of dairy, poultry, eggs, and fatty Coldwater fish rich in omega-3-fatty acid, seafood, occasional red meat, and some red wine

Melanoma: Begins in skin melanocytes with a good prognosis if found and treated early. How it looks? Larger than a pencil eraser, multi-colored—red, blue, purple, an irregular border, or growing in size.

Metabolic Syndrome: Syndrome X, the combination of high blood pressure, diabetes, central obesity, and abnormal lipids.

Methadone: a liquid opioid reducing the symptoms of withdrawal from drugs like heroin but without mood altering side effects. It may be used to enhance other pain meds.

MICD: Areco-occurring Mental Illness and Chemical Dependency.

Mild Cognitive Decline: A stage of mental change in men over 60. Expected decline of aging that may lead to further decline including problems with memory, language, thinking, and judgment.

Missionary Position: The sexual position when the man and woman are face-to- face.

 Moe's Dissection: The Piece-by-piece excision under microscopic guidance to a cancer-free edge of a squamous or basal cell skin cancer.

 Monosaturated Fats: The "Good Fat," are healthy fats found in olive oil, avocados, and certain nuts. They help with weight loss, reduce the risk of heart disease, and decrease inflammation.

Multiple Myeloma: A cancer of the plasma cells damaging bones, the immune system, the kidneys, and red cell production.

Muscle Mass: Comprises skeletal, smooth, and cardiac muscle, 84% in men 60-79.

My Plate: www.dietaryguidelines.gov. MyPlate A diet plan modulating eating habits emphasizing a variety of fruits, vegetables, grains, protein, including fortified soy alternatives.

Nautilus: Prototype isokinetic exercise machine that isolates specific muscle groups to adjustable safely controlled resistance and relaxation.

Neuroleptic: Antipsychotics, are psychotropic medications to manage psychoses, such as schizophrenia and are the mainstay often with mood stabilizers in the treatment of bipolar disorders.

NICU: Neurological Intensive Care Unit: Monitors traumatic brain injury (TBI).

Nordic Track: Simple exercise device simulating classic (striding) movements of two sliding boards (skis) and simultaneous poling (pullies).

Nutrient Dense Foods: Includes foods like kale, learn meats, whole grains, nuts, seeds, beans, and peas.

Okinawan Diet: Emphasizing soy products, fish, seaweed. Consistent with the lowest levels of cardiovascular disease.

Oral Sex: Mutual oral pleasuring by either or both sexes as a primary way to achieve orgasm or as foreplay to intercourse.

Oral Squamous Cancer: 84% survival rate with early detection.

Orgasm: The climax of sexual excitement characterized by feelings of intense pleasure in the genitals and body culminating in ejaculation.

Oropharynx: The part of the pharynx lying between the soft palate and the hyroid bone.

Overload Resistance Training: Progressive resistance weight training of increasing weights for sequential sets.

Osteoarthritis: Cartilage destruction at the ends of bones like the knees and hips, hands, neck, and lower back that worsens over time with morning stiffness, and evolving pain is the most common symptom.

Osteopenia: Less than normal bone density.

Osteoporosis: Compromised bone density with increased porosity, diminished density, and brittle bone resulting in bone damage.

Oxygenation: Oxygenation is the process of oxygen diffusing passively from the alveolus to the pulmonary capillaries, where it binds to hemoglobin in red blood cells or dissolves into the plasma. Insufficient oxygenation is termed hypoxemia.

Pancreatic Cancer: A cancer associated with weight loss, abdominal pain, and especially in men over 70 has a five-year survival rate of 7%.

Periodontal Disease: Gum infection that can lead to tooth and bone destruction and prevented by brushing and flossing.

Pescatarian: A vegetarian who eats fish.

Pharynx: The mucous membrane-lined space behind the nose and mouth connecting to the esophagus.

Plyometrics: Rapid and quick bursts of movement enhancing speed.

Pneumonia: Infection of the interstitial tissue and air sacs of the lung.

Polypill: Physical aerobic activity and a well-balanced diet to increase and maintain fitness.

Post menopause: After 12 months without a period during which women may experience hot flashes, vaginal dryness, sleep, and mood changes.

Prefrontal cortex: Responsible for reward, emotion, and motivation. The dorsal (dPFC) controls higher cognitive function and executive function.

Presarcopenia: Low muscle mass without the weakness of sarcopenia.

Proprioception: Our "sixth sense: Body awareness sensed by proprioceptors located in muscles and joints in our lower extremities and controlling force and speed of movement, maintaining muscle tone and balance.

PSA: Prostate Specific Antigen: Prostate cancer screen. Begin at 50 or earlier if high risk (African Americans or family history) until age 70, or as a screen for relapse from prostate cancer.

Pseudodementia: A similar presentation of dementia but usually reversible with appropriate adjustment of medications.

Psychiatrist: A medical doctor who prescribes psychotropics.

Psychologist: A counsellor with a masters or doctorate degree who performs testing and/or therapy for assisting mental health.

Pubococcygeal Muscles: Forms the pelvic floor (hammock). Assists with urination and contracts in orgasm.

PUD: Peptic ulcer disease caused by Heliobacter pylori (H. Pylori)

Pulse Pressure: Systolic minus diastolic blood pressures. Widens with age with loss of compliance of the muscular lining of arterial blood vessels.

Pyelonephritis: A serious kidney infection as a progression of urethritis or cystitis (of the bladder.

Prostatic hypertrophy(BPH): Common age-related increase in prostate size that can adversely affect urination with frequency, hesitancy, and incomplete emptying.

Pseudodementia: Not a diagnosis of neurological degeneration such as dementia, but can be caused by depression.

Quadriceps: "QUADS" Hefty hip flexors on the front of the thigh and opposed by the hamstrings (Biceps Femoris).

Radical Prostatectomy: Complete removal of the prostate, seminal vessels, some lymph glands, often in conjunction with radiation, chemotherapy, and immunotherapy for cancer.

Red Lining: Pushing exercise to maximal aerobic capacity called the anaerobic threshold or VO_{max}

Renal Failure: When the kidneys lose their ability to remove waste and balance fluids. Creatinine, muscle breakdown product, rises frequently with blood urea nitrogen (BUN).

Retinopathy: Destruction of the small vessels behind the retina at the back of the eye from hypertension or diabetes damaging the macula, the center of vision.

Rotator Cuff Damage: Either partial or complete tearing of suprascapularis, subscapularis, teres minor or major. Amenable to physical therapy or surgery.

SAD: Seasonal affective disorder experienced by some in sunless seasons that can be improved with light therapy at 10,000 lux for 30-45 minutes a day.

SA Node: Sinoatrial node initiates electrical conduction from the right atrium beginning contraction of the heart and innervating the AV node above the ventricles.

Sarcopenia: The accelerated loss of skeletal muscle mass of aging accompanied by falls, functional decline, frailty, and mortality.

Saturated Fats: Single-bonded glycerides, primarily animal fats high in LDL cholesterol.

SCARP: Story, Categorization, Association, Repetition, Picture: a great mnemonic to enhance aging memory or after traumatic brain injury(TBI). *Eric*

Seizures: Potentially life-threatening grand mal, lesser petite mal, or the absence variety associated with irregular electrical brain activity.

Seminal vesicles: Two glands behind the bladder secreting fluid that compose semen.

Silver and Fit and Silver Sneakers: Two gym memberships available with certain supplemental insurance plans.

Slow Twitch Muscle Fibers: Muscle fibres predominant in endurance activities of greater quantity in men over 60.

Small Cell Lung Cancer: Bronchial "Oat" cell occurs more in men over 60. It is smoking-related and in advanced form, has an 8% survival rate.

Squamous Carcinoma: With basal cell carcinoma, the most common skin cancer that is 100% curable. It is caused by excessive sun especially in lighter skinned individuals that presents as a crusty, scaling, bleeding, or itching skin blotch, especially in exposed areas of the face, ears, nose, and arms.

Spermicide: A contraceptive inserted into the vagina that kills active sperm advisedly used with barriers such as a condom, a diaphragm, or cervical cap. Alone it does not prevent STDs.

SSRIs: Serotonin reuptake inhibitors, the new generation of antidepressants used in the treatment of major depressive disorders that includes fluoxetine, citalopram, and others.

Stairmaster: A low impact aerobics step exercise machine.

Statins: Medication to lower low-density lipoproteins by blocking the enzyme in the liver that produces cholesterol. Statins enhance absorption of plaques in arteries, especially for those at high risk for developing cardiovascular disease with a LDL level over 190mg/dL.

STDs: Sexually transmitted diseases: chlamydia, gonorrhoea, syphilis, HIV, and others spread by vaginal, oral, and anal sexual activities.

Stent: Metal or plastic temporary or permanent tube placed in a blood vessel, canal, or duct to relieve obstruction.

Stretching: Movements to lengthen muscle fibrils and muscles.

Stroke Volume (SV): The volume of blood with each contraction of the left ventricle.

Stroke: Damage to brain tissue either from broken blood vessels or compromised circulation.

Subdural Hematoma: A dangerous increased pressure from an acute, subacute, or chronic brain bleed under the dura and skull and above the thin brain cover, known as a traumatic brain injury (TBI).

Suboxone: Medication that is the combination of buprenorphine and naloxone that is used in medication-assisted treatment(MAT) for opioid disorder to avoid withdrawal.

Substance Use Disorder (SUDS): Overuse, abuse, or dependence of, legal or illegal narcotics.

Systolic Blood Pressure: Upper of the two pressure measurements of blood pressure. Generally, increases in men over 60 as compliance and elasticity of arterioles decreases.

Tachycardia: Heart rate over 100.

Tendon: Flexible but inelastic cord made of fibrous collagen attaching muscle to bone and more frequently than muscle ruptured in men over 60.

Testes (Balls): Two glands in the scrotum that produce sperm and testosterone.

Testosterone: Male hormone that enhances sperm production, hair pattern, sexual drive that gradually diminishes in men over 60.

Transient Ischemic Attack (TIA): A temporary and reversible mini stroke at risk for becoming a completed stroke. It can include weakness on one or both sides of the body, vision problems, or slurred speech.

Type 1 Diabetes: Juvenile diabetes. Insulin dependent and associated with metabolic acidosis.

Type 2 Diabetes: Maturity-onset, obesity-related, and hereditary.

Triglycerides: A triglyceride is an ester derived from glycerol and three fatty acids. Triglycerides are the main constituents of body fat in humans and other vertebrates.

Thallium scan: See Cardiolite Test.

Traumatic Brain Syndrome: Major cause of death and disability from head injury and includes concussions.

Tricyclic Antidepressants: Block brain reabsorption of neurotransmitters, serotonin and norepinephrine, but complicated by drowsiness and urinary retention, greater suicide risk by overdose of life-threatening rhythm disturbances. Include Elavil (amitriptyline), Sinequan (doxepin), and Tofranil (imipramine).

Ultraviolet Light Protective Clothing: UPF 50 woven fabric blocks 98% of both UVA and UVB rays.

Urethra: The tube between the bladder and urinary meatus traversing the prostate and closed by the urethral sphincter that is the conduit for both urine and sperm, and with prostatic hypertrophy may become gradually compromised.

Vascular Dementia (VaD): Cognitive difficulty with reasoning and judgment. In later stages, memory is affected particularly in those at higher risk of stroke due to obesity or diabetes.

Vas deferens: Ducts transport sperm from the epididymis around the tests to the ejaculatory ducts in anticipation of orgasm and ejaculation.

Vasoconstriction: The constriction of muscular arteries as in hypothermia.

Vasodilator: A blood pressure medication that relaxes and opens smooth muscles including ACE inhibitors (angiotensin converting enzyme), ARBs (angiotensin receptor blockers), nitroglycerine containing compounds (isosorbide dinitrate) for angina, hydralazine, calcium channel blockers, diuretics, and beta blockers.

Vegan: Someone who eats no animal products.

Vegetarian Diet: Someone who eats no animal meat with or without fish but may eat milk and eggs.

Ventricular Hypertrophy (LVH): Thickened cardiac muscle of the left ventricular chamber that can be the result of aortic stenosis, high blood pressure, or decades of endurance activity that can lead to rhythm disturbances and/or to heart failure.

Vertigo: Dizziness and imbalance primarily from malfunction of the semi-circular canals of the inner ear.

Vestibular System: Includes the semi-circular canals containing tiny bones (otoliths) in the inner ear and responsible for balance, orientation, and coordination.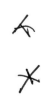

Viagra(sildenafil): The popular medication that relaxes the muscles of the smaller muscular arterioles of the penis and increases blood flow for engorgement. Note: avoid if on cardiac medications for angina containing nitrates.

Vitamin E: An antioxidant protecting against destructive free radicals.

$VO_{2\,max}$: Considered genetic and improved with specific training. It is the point of the shift from aerobic to anaerobic metabolism and before the sometimes painful accumulation of lactic acid.

Vulva: Female secondary sex organs that include the clitoris, labia major and minor, urinary meatus, vaginal opening, an initial hymen membrane, and secretory glands.

Water Pill: A diuretic that enhances urination and by decreasing blood volume lowers blood pressure. An example is hydrochlorothiazide.

Wheezing: A loud and prolonged raspy sound on a forced hard expiration is common in someone with asthma and, if appropriately treated, is reversible.

Widow Maker: Blockage of the left anterior descending artery (LAD) from the left coronary artery that can be lethal.

Zygoma: The bone that forms the prominence of the cheek (cheekbone) formed by the connection of the zygomatic and temporal bones.

Index

237

239

240

242

CPSIA information can be obtained
at www.ICGtesting.com
Printed in the USA
JSHW040327100323
38731JS00003B/9